Sandbag Fitness: 150 High Intensity Workouts

© Matthew Palfrey 2015

All rights reserved. No part of this book may be reproduced or transmitted in any form or by any means without written permission of the author.

Images by Alison Crocker

Original design by Will Slater

First Edition

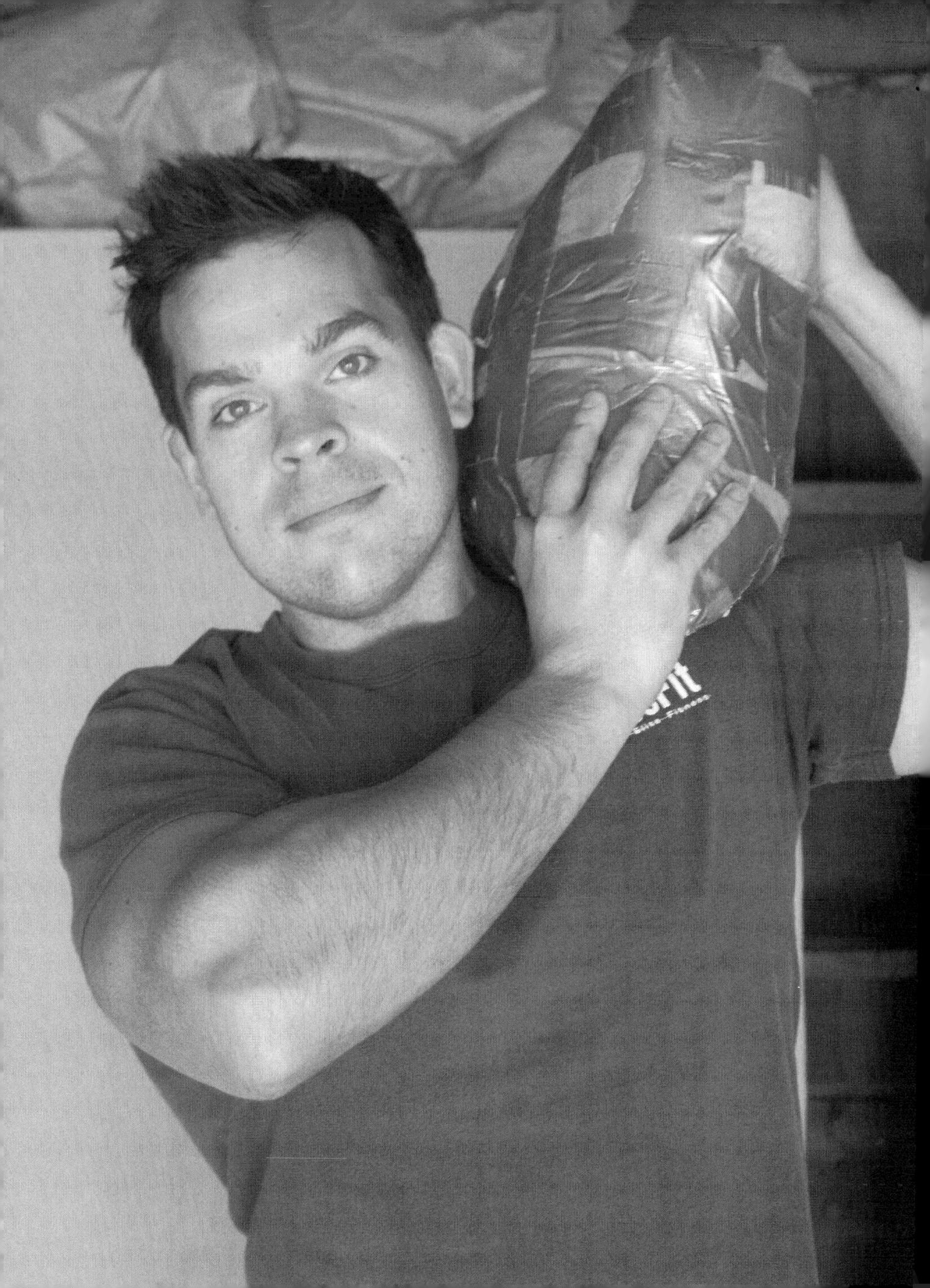

CONTENTS

CHAPTERS	PAGE
Disclaimer	4
Introduction	7
Part 1 - Training Basics	9-17
Part 2 - Strength Workouts	18-31
Part 3 - Endurance Workouts	32-55
Part 4 - Power Workouts	56-69
Part 5 - Agility Workouts	70-83
Part 6 - Upper Body Workouts	84-97
Part 7 - Lower Body Workouts	98-111
Part 8 - Simple Workouts	112-135
Part 9 - Running Workouts	136-149
Part 10 - Team Workouts	150-163
Part 11 - Quick Workouts	164-187
Part 12 - Sandbag-Only Workouts	188-201
Part 13 - Challenge Workouts	202-215
FAQ	218
Want To Learn More?	220
Acknowledgements	222
Notes	223

DISCLAIMER

Sandbag Fitness: 150 High Intensity Workouts is not meant to diagnose or treat any medical condition. It is designed as a resource for individuals to improve their general health and fitness. Individuals with any preexisting medical conditions should check with their doctor/physician before commencing any programme of physical activity.

The author cannot be held responsible for any injury, ill health or medical complication resulting from the use or misuse of this guide or any of the information contain herein. If you are unsure about its suitability for you, always check with a medical professional first.

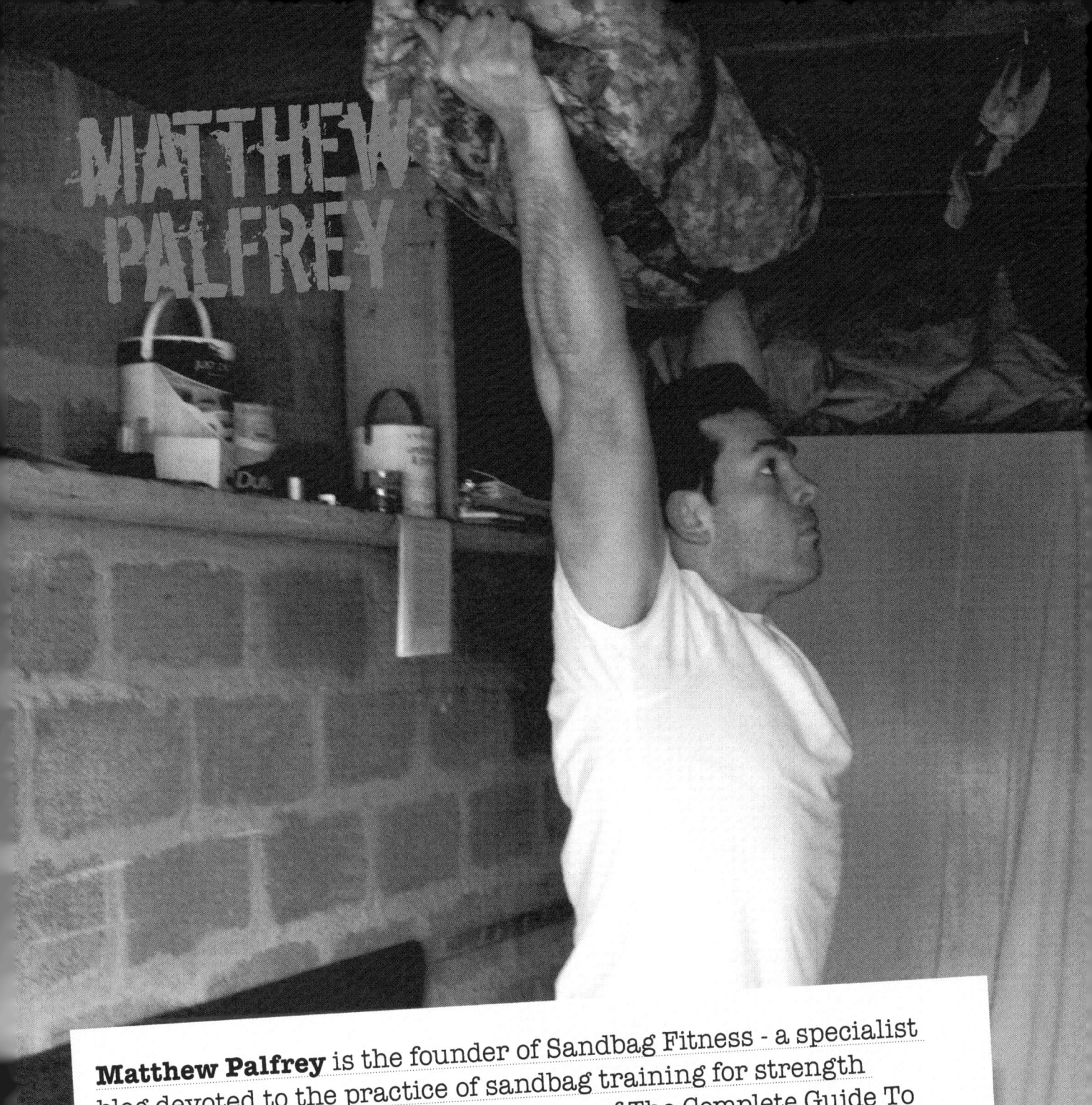

Matthew Palfrey is the founder of Sandbag Fitness - a specialist blog devoted to the practice of sandbag training for strength and conditioning. He is also the author of The Complete Guide To Sandbag Training, Sandbag Training For MMA & Combat Sports, Sandbag Fitness: Lean & Strong and the cofounder of Brute Force Europe.

Widely regarded as a leading expert in the field of sandbag training, Matthew writes for a number of publications including Onnit, EliteFTS and T-Nation.

SANDBAG FITNESS

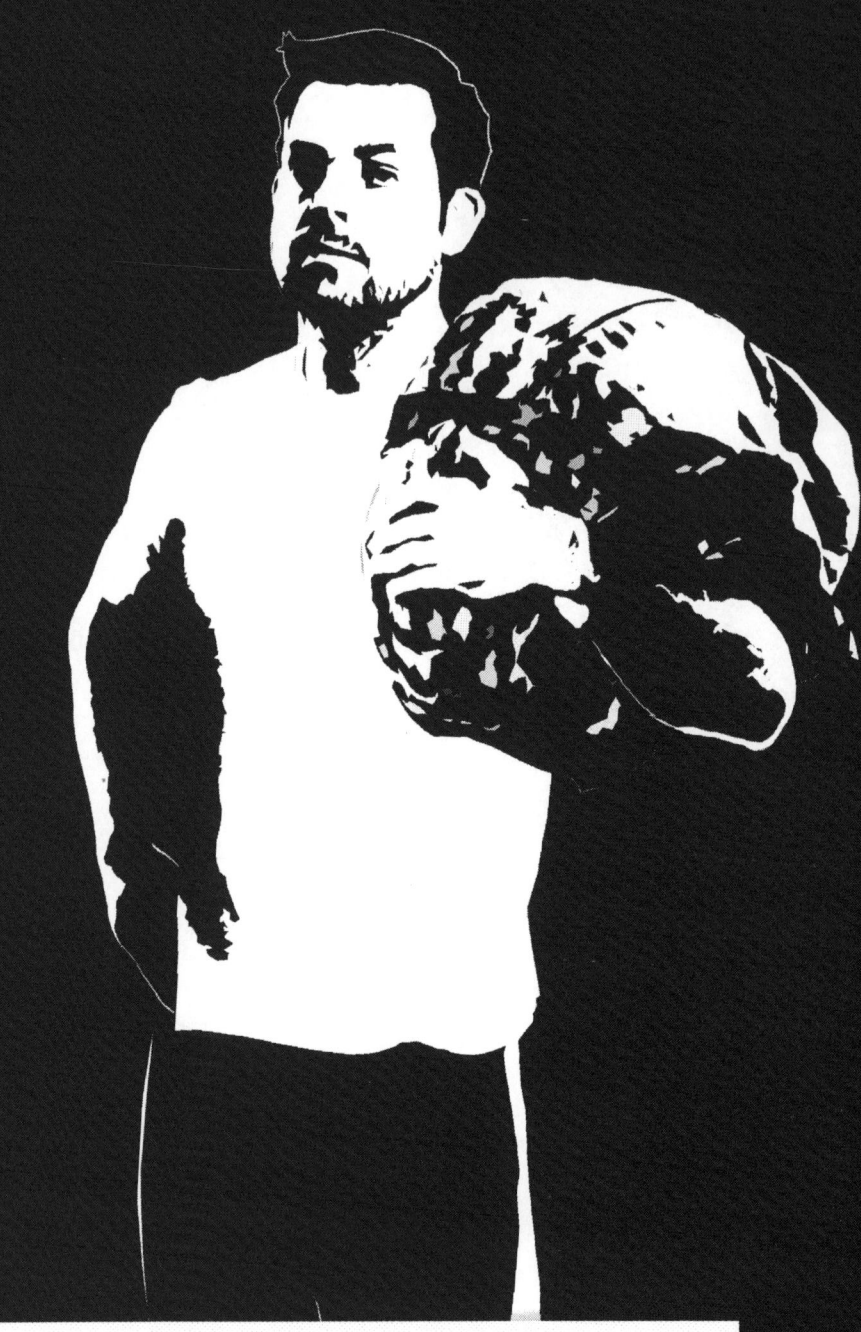

Sandbag Fitness is the no nonsense fitness company dedicated to the promotion and practice of sandbag training. They provide training information, sandbag training books and products, and support for anyone who wants to improve their strength, conditioning and general health.

For regular sandbag training workouts follow the Sandbag Fitness Blog.

Learn more: www.sandbagfitnessstore.com

INTRODUCTION

Sandbag Fitness: 150 High Intensity Workouts is a simple guide that has been written to provide you with a variety of different workout options. These have all been designed with broad goals in mind - like Strength, Endurance, Power and Agility. But, despite a general theme for each section of workouts there is one constant throughout - good quality, high intensity exercise sessions.

Like all good training programmes, there is no one-size-fits-all solution. You can use the workouts here to help build your sandbag training programme. Alternatively you might just want a pick up and go list of sandbag training workouts. Either way, I hope this guide is useful to you.

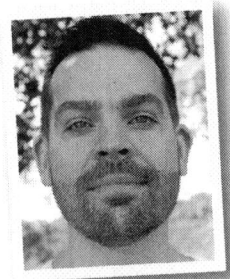
From the early days of the Sandbag Fitness Blog followers have been telling me that they loved my simple approach to training sessions. Thousands of people worldwide come to the blog on a weekly basis to get sandbag training workouts to follow. My ethos has always been to provide straightforward, challenging and effective training sessions that everyone can benefit from. I truly believe that fitness training does not need to be complicated to be effective.

So this guide is just that. A very simple breakdown of some of the workouts that I've developed over the years, all categorised to make it easier to choose the right one for you. But although it's simple, don't misinterpret that for basic. There is a huge amount of content here to get through but this is not a book of light bedtime reading. The only learning here comes from dusting off your training shoes, loading up that sandbag and getting a score in the book for every single workout.

So what are you waiting for?

Train hard!

Matt
Sandbag Fitness

PART 1
TRAINING BASICS

Part 1: Training Basics

WHAT YOU NEED FOR THIS PROGRAM

Sandbag training is a simple thing and you do not need to invest a huge amount of money or time in anything before getting started. In fact, getting started is by far the most important thing you can do. That being said, there are a few pieces of equipment that will make your sessions more effective.

If some of my recommendations are outside of your budget then don't worry about it. I'm not one of those coaches who'll bully you into buying something by saying "If you were really serious you'd find the money to buy these things…" Instead, I give recommendations for free/homemade alternatives to all of the equipment suggested here. So the only real commitment is that you need to work hard and stay focused. Rarely is your access to good quality equipment the deciding factor in your success or failure.

HOMEMADE SANDBAGS

When I began sandbag training I started with a homemade sandbag. It's a great option if you're on a tight budget or want to try out the training method before investing in it.

By far and away the simplest way to construct a homemade sandbag is by using a duffel bag or holdall. You can then add contractor/builders bags of sand directly into this outer shell. These bags of sand are generally sold in 55lb weights so you may need to adjust the weight before you can start. To do this, make a small slit in the bag of sand and remove what you don't need. You'll then need to tape up the bag to avoid any leakage (use strong tape for this).

One of the major issues with this method is that you will also need to think about how to add weight to the sandbag as you improve your strength, power and conditioning. A simple way around this is to make a number of smaller sandbags that you can add into the outer shell when you need to. Ziploc bags filled with around 2-4lbs of sand work well (and use tape liberally to seal). Alternatively, you might want to make a range of different sized sandbags and then choose the appropriate one for each session.

CUSTOM MADE SANDBAGS

Brute Force Sandbags make the worlds toughest sandbags for strength and conditioning. Brute Force make the Sandbag Fitness range of products and we sell a range of their sandbags in our online store.

The major advantages of using a custom-made sandbag like this are:

- It comes with internal filler bags, making it easy to change the weight of the sandbag when you need to
- It is built to last and will not split, even under the toughest abuse
- The inclusion of handles on the sandbag make it easier to complete exercises like rows and Deadlifts

To purchase sandbags please visit www.sandbagfitnessstore.com

TIMER

All good programmes are measurable so you'll need a way to time some of your workouts and rest periods. This is particularly important as it will give you a baseline with which to gauge improvements over time. And without some aspect of measurement you may find yourself going through the motions.

Nowadays, most people have access to a timer of some variety already, perhaps through their watch or phone. But if you want to purchase an exercises timer that suits the sandbag training sessions in this guide then I recommend a Gymboss Timer. I use one myself for my interval training sessions.

To purchase a Gymboss Timer please visit www.gymboss.com

PULL UP BAR

You don't need anything too complex to perform things like Pull Ups, Hanging Knee Raises and Toes-to-Bar. If you don't have access to a bar with which to perform some of the hanging exercises then there are lots of ways to improvise.

Tree branches, suspension trainers, gymnastic rings or climbing frames are all viable options. Just make sure that whatever you use is safe enough to support your weight.

SKIPPING ROPE

A speed rope can be useful but anything is sufficient. Skipping ropes tend to be very inexpensive and they are a great addition to the training programmes in ths guide, and as a general means to warm-up and build endurance and agility.

BOX/STEP/BENCH

You'll need some type of sturdy box, step or platform on which to perform things like Sandbag Step Ups, Box Jumps and Sandbag Hip Thrusts. If you don't have access to a custom box or bench then I know lots of people who have constructed their own box for these purposes.

Alternatively, a park bench, wall or stacked boxes can serve the purpose quite well. Again, just be sure that whatever you are using can stand up to any loading that you'll put it under.

For the purposes of this programme a box or step approximately 24 inches high is perfect.

HOW TO FOLLOW THE WORKOUTS

Once you've chosen a workout to tackle you'll find each one divided into 4 distinct sections. These will provide information regarding that specific workout and also give you some targets to aim for. But, despite the targets described, remember that you can always make any of the workouts easier or harder. Adjusting the weight, intensity of the exercise or overall volume can always be used as a technique for making the workout more appropriate for you.

- Workout - detailing the specific exercises, required repetitions and sets for the workout
- Measurement - detailing how you should record your performance for that workout
- Target - detailing the recommended sandbag weight, time or repetitions required
- Performance - use this diary section to record your performance each time you go through the workout

TRACKING

One of the key factors in making progress with your fitness training programme is tracking, or measurement. While I think that working out for the sake of it has some merit, my experience is that a specific target always helps to improve performance.

Whatever your overall goal, tracking your performance gives you something tangible to work towards. Without this you may find yourself going through the motions. What should you be working towards? Going 1 second faster, adding 1 repetition, adding 1lb of extra sand to your bag. These are all small, achievable incremental improvements that everyone can make. The Measurement and Target sections in each workout will also make it clear exactly what you should be aiming for.

I urge you to utilise the performance section at the bottom of each workout page. For the avoidance of doubt, I consider this book only "done" if you manage to complete all 150 workouts five times, ideally showing some improvement in subsequent attempts.

That's a total of 750 sandbag training workouts, or around 5 years if you complete an average of 3 per week. Are you up to the challenge?

Of course, numerical measurement like this is only part of the overall picture. While it will give you an indicator of your general progress it does not replace common sense, good technique or your intrinsic feeling of improvement.

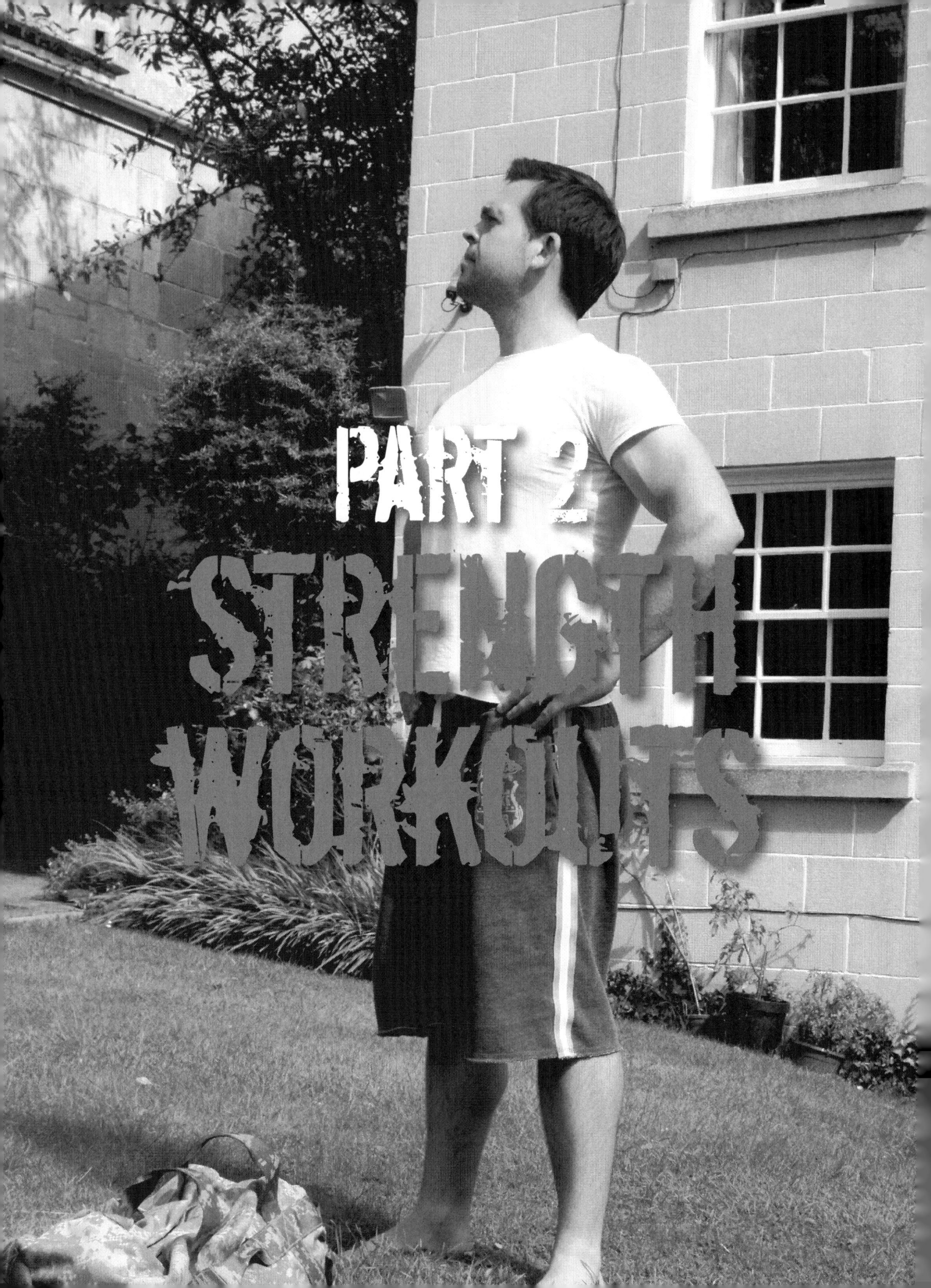

PART 2
STRENGTH WORKOUTS

Strength

noun | stren(k)th

1. The quality or state of being physically strong.
2. The ability to resist being moved or broken by a force.
3. The quality that allows someone to deal with problems in a determined and effective way.

Use these workouts to build, develop and maintain your physical strength.

The workouts in this section are focused on compound exercises like Squats, Deadlifts, Presses and Pulls. When working on strength development the key is making sure you have enough weight in your sandbag, not being afraid to have extended rest periods between sets, and working hard for each and every lift.

STRENGTH

"I LOVE TO LIFT HEAVY SANDBAGS. I FIND THAT SANDBAG LIFTING BUILDS A TYPE OF RUGGED, TOTAL BODY STRENGTH THAT IS IMPOSSIBLE TO DUPLICATE WITH OTHER EQUIPMENT."

BROOKS KUBRIK

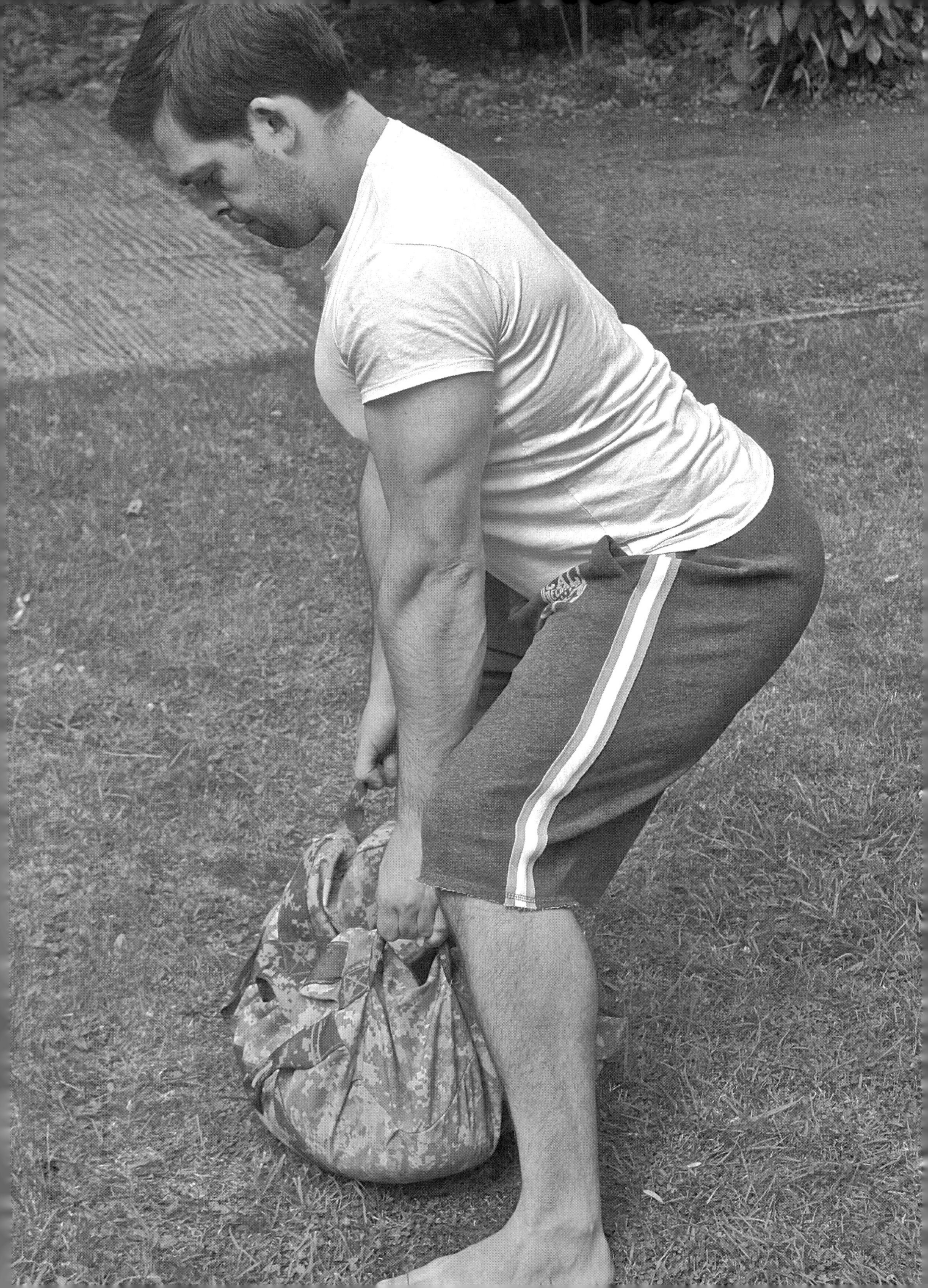

Part 2: Strength Workouts

#1 STRENGTH

WORKOUT

20 Sandbag Clean & Press

MEASUREMENT

Aim to complete the workout in as fast a time as you can. Record this time, and the sandbag weight used.

TARGET WEIGHT

Aim for a sandbag weighing 75% of your bodyweight

Date					
Reps/ Weight/ Time/ Rounds					

#2 STRENGTH

WORKOUT

Perform a single Sandbag Power Clean and Sandbag Push Jerk. Then, lower the sandbag across your shoulders and perform Sandbag Back Squats to failure, to finish each set.

MEASUREMENT

Rest for 2 - 4 minutes between rounds and repeat for 5 rounds in total.

Record your total number of Sandbag Back Squat repetitions, and the sandbag weight used.

TARGET WEIGHT

Aim for a sandbag weighing 75% of your bodyweight

Date					
Reps/ Weight/ Time/ Rounds					

#3 STRENGTH

WORKOUT

Max Sandbag Front Squats
Max Pull Ups

Rest for 2 - 4 minutes and repeat for a total of 5 rounds.

MEASUREMENT

Record your total number of Sandbag Back Squat and Pull Up repetitions, and the sandbag weight used.

TARGET WEIGHT

Aim for a sandbag weighing 75% of your bodyweight

Date					
Reps/ Weight/ Time/ Rounds					

… # #4 STRENGTH

WORKOUT

5 Sandbag Clean
5 Sandbag Push Jerk
5 Sandbag Back Squat

Rest for 2 - 4 minutes and repeat for a total of 5 rounds.

MEASUREMENT

Aim to lift as much weight as you can during this workout. Record your time, and the sandbag weight used.

TARGET WEIGHT

Aim for a sandbag weighing 75% of your bodyweight

Date					
Reps/ Weight/ Time/ Rounds					

#5 STRENGTH

WORKOUT

10 Sandbag Cleans
10 Sandbag Overhead Press
10 Sandbag Back Squats
10 Sandbag Floor Press

Rest for 1 - 2 minutes and repeat for a total of 5 rounds.

MEASUREMENT

Aim to lift as much weight as you can during this workout. Record your time, and the sandbag weight used.

TARGET WEIGHT

Aim for a sandbag weighing 75% of your bodyweight

Date					
Reps/ Weight/ Time/ Rounds					

#6 STRENGTH

WORKOUT

10 Sandbag Bear Hug Squats
30 Push Ups

As many rounds as possible in 15 minutes.

MEASUREMENT

Record the number of rounds you can complete in 15 minutes. Record the weight of the sandbag you used to complete this workout.

TARGET WEIGHT

Aim for a sandbag weighing 75% of your bodyweight

Date					
Reps/ Weight/ Time/ Rounds					

#7 STRENGTH

WORKOUT

5 Sandbag Bear Hug Squats
5 Sandbag Overhead Press
20m Sandbag Load Carry

Rest for 2 - 4 minutes and repeat for a total of 5 rounds.

MEASUREMENT

Aim to lift as much weight as you can during this workout. Record your time, and the sandbag weight used.

TARGET WEIGHT

Aim for a sandbag weighing 75% of your body weight

Date					
Reps/ Weight/ Time/ Rounds					

#8 STRENGTH

WORKOUT

5 Sandbag Zercher Squats
5 Sandbag Floor Press
5 Sandbag Shoulder Get Ups (each side)

Rest for 2 - 4 minutes and repeat for a total of 5 rounds.

MEASUREMENT

Aim to lift as much weight as you can during this workout. Record your time, and the sandbag weight used.

TARGET WEIGHT

Aim for a sandbag weighing 75% of your body weight

Date					
Reps/ Weight/ Time/ Rounds					

#9 STRENGTH

WORKOUT

Max Sandbag Zercher Squats
Max Sandbag Overhead Press
Max Pull Ups

Rest for 2 - 4 minutes and repeat for a total of 5 rounds.

MEASUREMENT

Record the total number of repetitions, and the sandbag weight used.

TARGET WEIGHT

Aim for a sandbag weighing 75% of your body weight

Date					
Reps/ Weight/ Time/ Rounds					

#10 STRENGTH

WORKOUT

5 Sandbag Shoulder Get Ups (each side)
Max Pull Ups

Rest for 2 - 4 minutes and repeat for a total of 5 rounds.

MEASUREMENT

Record the total number of Pull Up repetitions, and the sandbag weight used.

TARGET WEIGHT

Aim for a sandbag weighing 75% of your body weight

Date					
Reps/ Weight/ Time/ Rounds					

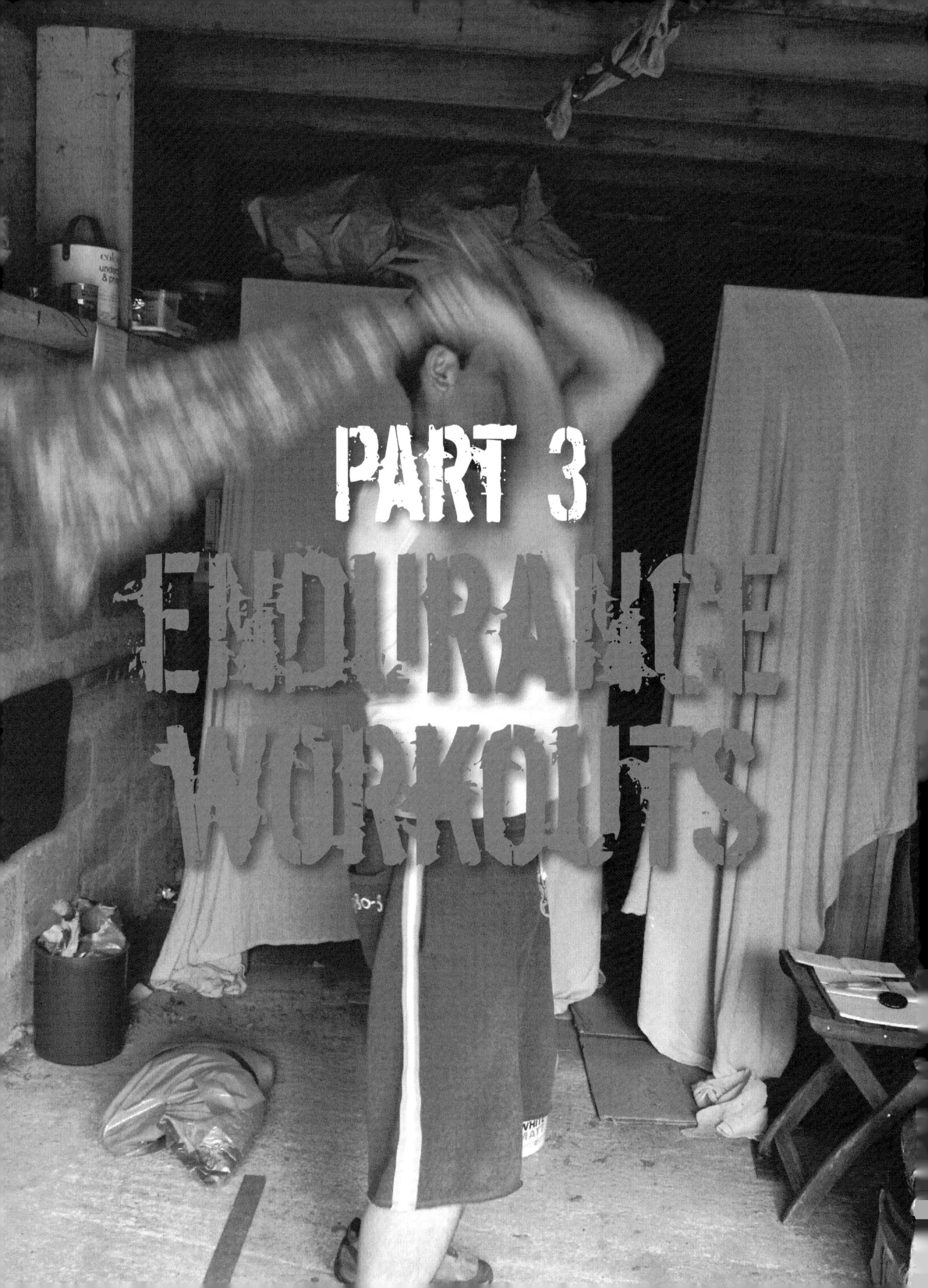

PART 3
ENDURANCE WORKOUTS

Endurance

noun | en·dur·ance

1. The ability to do something difficult for a long time.
2. The ability to deal with pain or suffering that continues for a long time.
3. The quality of continuing for a long time.

Use these workouts to build, develop and maintain your endurance.

You'll typically find that these workouts stress higher repetitions and lighter weights, and generally speaking they won't have any specific rest periods. When working on your endurance the key is selecting an appropriate weight for the workout, being selective with micro-breaks, and keeping focused on the end goal.

ENDURANCE

"You can hurt more than you ever thought possible, then continue until you discover that hurting isn't that big a deal."

— SCOTT JUREK

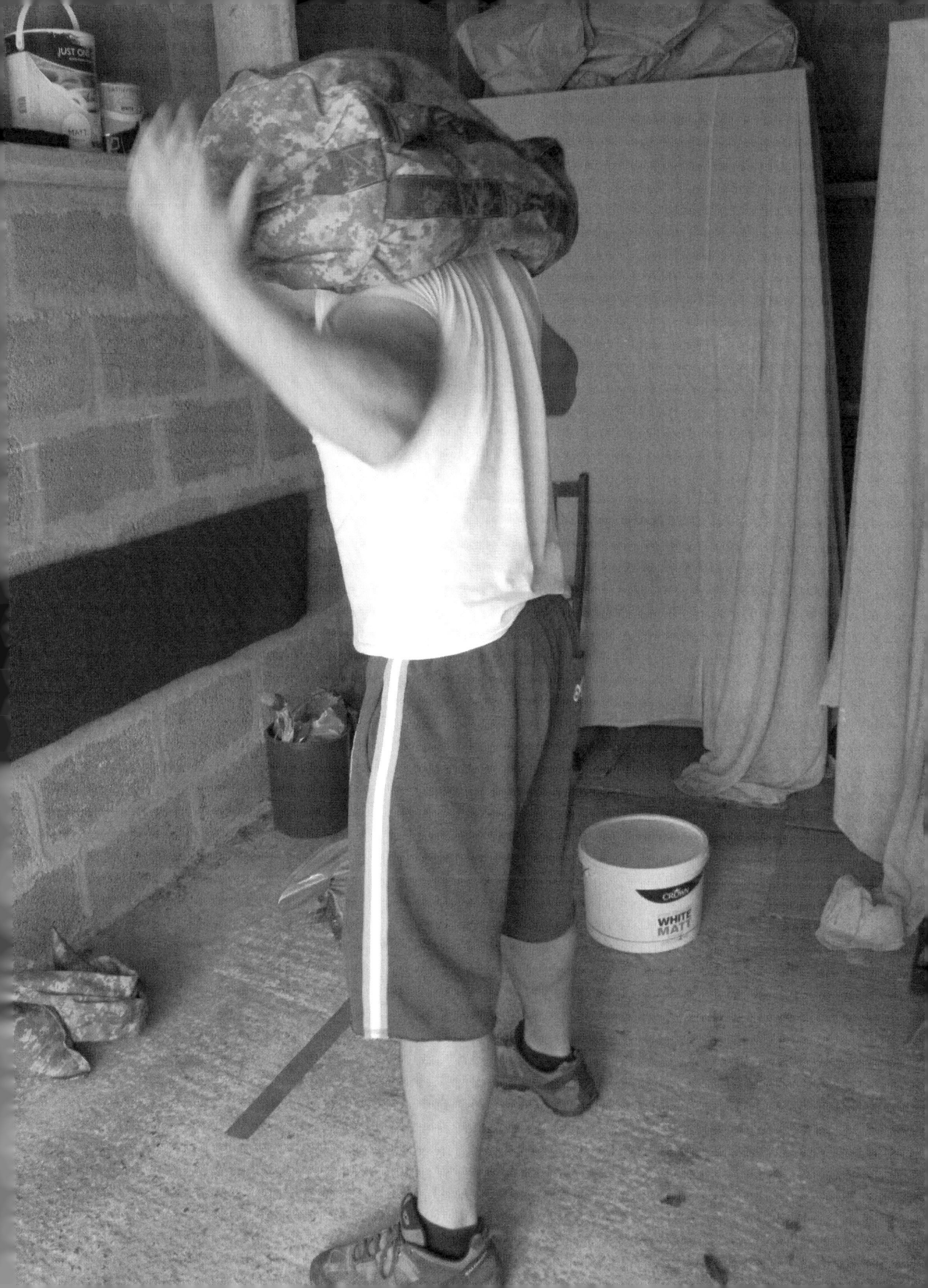

#1 ENDURANCE

WORKOUT

20 Sandbag Round-the-Worlds (10 in each direction)
10 Sandbag High Pulls
10 Sandbag Zercher Squats
10 Sandbag Overhead Presses

Repeat for a total of 5 rounds.

MEASUREMENT

Aim to complete the workout in as fast a time as you can. Record the weight of the sandbag you used to complete this workout.

TARGET WEIGHT

Aim for a sandbag weighing 30% of your body weight, 15% for the Sandbag Round-the-Worlds

Date					
Reps/ Weight/ Time/ Rounds					

#2 ENDURANCE

WORKOUT

22 Box Jumps
22 Sandbag Push Jerks
22 Sandbag Zercher Squats

Repeat for a total of 6 rounds.

MEASUREMENT

Aim to complete the workout in as fast a time as you can. Record the weight of the sandbag you used to complete this workout.

TARGET WEIGHT

Aim for a sandbag weighing 30% of your body weight

Date					
Reps/ Weight/ Time/ Rounds					

#3 ENDURANCE

WORKOUT

100 Sandbag Shoulder Squats (switch shoulders as you wish)
100 Sandbag Push Jerks
100 Sandbag Cleans
100 Pull Ups

Complete as fast as you can and in any order you wish - reps can be broken up into sets.

MEASUREMENT

Aim to complete the workout in as fast a time as you can. Record the weight of the sandbag you used to complete this workout.

TARGET WEIGHT

Aim for a sandbag weighing 30% of your body weight

Date					
Reps/ Weight/ Time/ Rounds					

#4 ENDURANCE

WORKOUT

15 - 1 of the following exercises (perform 15 repetitions of each one, then 14 etc.):

Sandbag Floor Press
Sandbag Shoulder Get Ups (switch shoulders between rounds)
Sandbag Zercher Squats
Sandbag High Pulls

MEASUREMENT

Aim to complete the workout in as fast a time as you can. Record the weight of the sandbag you used to complete this workout.

TARGET WEIGHT

Aim for a sandbag weighing 30% of your body weight

Date					
Reps/ Weight/ Time/ Rounds					

#5 ENDURANCE

WORKOUT

5 Pull Ups
10 Sandbag Push Press
15 Sandbag Shoulder Squats (change shoulder each round)

Complete as many rounds as possible in 20 minutes.

MEASUREMENT

Record the number of rounds you can complete in 20 minutes. Record the weight of the sandbag you used to complete this workout.

TARGET WEIGHT

Aim for a sandbag weighing 40% of your body weight

Date					
Reps/ Weight/ Time/ Rounds					

#6 ENDURANCE

WORKOUT

50 Sandbag Front Squats
50 Sandbag Overhead Presses
50 Sandbag Cleans

Repeat for a total of 3 rounds.

MEASUREMENT

Aim to complete the workout in as fast a time as you can. Record the weight of the sandbag you used to complete this workout.

TARGET WEIGHT

Aim for a sandbag weighing 40% of your body weight

Date					
Reps/ Weight/ Time/ Rounds					

Part 3: Endurance Workouts

#7 ENDURANCE

WORKOUT

Box Jumps, Sandbag Cleans, Sandbag Front Squats, Sit Ups, Sandbag Push Jerks.

Perform each exercise for 1 minute, giving a total round of 5 minutes. Record the number of repetitions performed within each minute for each exercise. There is a 1 minute rest period between each set of 5 exercises but a running clock during each round. Repeat for 3 rounds in total.

MEASUREMENT

Record your total repetitions for the whole sequence. Record the weight of the sandbag you used to complete this workout.

TARGET WEIGHT

Aim for a sandbag weighing 30% of your body weight

Date					
Reps/ Weight/ Time/ Rounds					

#8 ENDURANCE

WORKOUT

10 Sandbag High Pulls
10 Push Ups
10 Sandbag Goblet Squats
10 Sandbag Overhead Press

Repeat for a total of 5 rounds.

MEASUREMENT

Aim to complete the workout in as fast a time as you can. Record the weight of the sandbag you used to complete this workout.

TARGET WEIGHT

Aim for a sandbag weighing 30% of your body weight

Date					
Reps/ Weight/ Time/ Rounds					

#9 ENDURANCE

WORKOUT

100 Sandbag Thruster Burpees
150 Pull Ups

Complete as fast as you can and in any order you wish - reps can be broken up into sets.

MEASUREMENT

Aim to complete the workout in as fast a time as you can. Record the weight of the sandbag you used to complete this workout.

TARGET WEIGHT

Aim for a sandbag weighing 30% of your body weight

Date					
Reps/ Weight/ Time/ Rounds					

#10 ENDURANCE

WORKOUT

200 Skips
20 Sandbag Back Squats
200 Skips
20 Sandbag Overhead Presses

Repeat for a total of 4 rounds.

MEASUREMENT

Aim to complete the workout in as fast a time as you can. Record the weight of the sandbag you used to complete this workout.

TARGET WEIGHT

Aim for a sandbag weighing 30% of your body weight

Date					
Reps/ Weight/ Time/ Rounds					

#11 ENDURANCE

WORKOUT

15 - 1 of the following exercises (perform 15 repetitions of each one, then 14 etc.):

Sandbag High Pulls
Sandbag Push Press
Sandbag Front Squats

MEASUREMENT

Aim to complete the workout in as fast a time as you can. Record the weight of the sandbag you used to complete this workout.

TARGET WEIGHT

Aim for a sandbag weighing 30% of your body weight

Date					
Reps/ Weight/ Time/ Rounds					

#12 ENDURANCE

WORKOUT

20 seconds of work, 10 seconds of rest - repeat for a total of 8 working intervals. No rest between exercises.

Toes-to-Bar
Sandbag Shoulder-to-Shoulder Press
Sandbag Bent-over-Row
Push Ups

MEASUREMENT

Record your total repetitions for the whole sequence. Record the weight of the sandbag you used to complete this workout.

TARGET WEIGHT

Aim for a sandbag weighing 40% of your body weight

Date					
Reps/ Weight/ Time/ Rounds					

Part 3: Endurance Workouts

#13 ENDURANCE

WORKOUT

100 Push Ups
100 Sandbag Zecher Squats
100 Sandbag High Pulls
100 Body weight Squats

Complete as fast as you can and in any order you wish - reps can be broken up into sets.

MEASUREMENT

Record your total repetitions for the whole sequence. Record the weight of the sandbag you used to complete this workout.

TARGET WEIGHT

Aim for a sandbag weighing 30% of your body weight

Date					
Reps/ Weight/ Time/ Rounds					

#14 ENDURANCE

WORKOUT

50 Sandbag Step Ups
50 Sandbag Shoulder-to-Shoulder Press
50 Sandbag Good Mornings

Repeat for a total of 4 rounds.

MEASUREMENT

Aim to complete the workout in as fast a time as you can. Record the weight of the sandbag you used to complete this workout.

TARGET WEIGHT

Aim for a sandbag weighing 30% of your body weight

Date					
Reps/ Weight/ Time/ Rounds					

#15 ENDURANCE

WORKOUT

20 - 1 of the following exercises (perform 20 repetitions of each one, then 19 etc.):

T-Push Ups
Sandbag Back Squats
Sandbag Deadlifts

MEASUREMENT

Aim to complete the workout in as fast a time as you can. Record the weight of the sandbag you used to complete this workout.

TARGET WEIGHT

Aim for a sandbag weighing 30% of your body weight

Date					
Reps/ Weight/ Time/ Rounds					

#16 ENDURANCE

WORKOUT

50 Body weight Squats
25 Sandbag Back Squats
50 Sandbag Walking Lunge (25 each side)
25 Sandbag Overhead Presses

Repeat for a total of 3 rounds.

MEASUREMENT

Aim to complete the workout in as fast a time as you can. Record the weight of the sandbag you used to complete this workout.

TARGET WEIGHT

Aim for a sandbag weighing 30% of your body weight

Date					
Reps/ Weight/ Time/ Rounds					

#17 ENDURANCE

WORKOUT

100m Sandbag Load Carry
30 Body weight Squats
20 Push Ups

Repeat for a total of 6 rounds.

MEASUREMENT

Aim to complete the workout in as fast a time as you can. Record the weight of the sandbag you used to complete this workout.

TARGET WEIGHT

Aim for a sandbag weighing 30% of your body weight

Date					
Reps/ Weight/ Time/ Rounds					

#18 ENDURANCE

WORKOUT

200m Sandbag Shoulder Load Carry
200m Sandbag Zercher Load Carry
200m Sandbag Overhead Load Carry
200m Sandbag Drag

MEASUREMENT

Aim to complete the workout in as fast a time as you can. Record the weight of the sandbag you used to complete this workout.

TARGET WEIGHT

Aim for a sandbag weighing 50% of your body weight

Date					
Reps/ Weight/ Time/ Rounds					

#19 ENDURANCE

WORKOUT

100m Sandbag Overhead Load Carry
20 Sandbag High Pulls
100 Skips

Repeat for a total of 10 rounds.

MEASUREMENT

Aim to complete the workout in as fast a time as you can. Record the weight of the sandbag you used to complete this workout.

TARGET WEIGHT

Aim for a sandbag weighing 30% of your body weight

Date					
Reps/ Weight/ Time/ Rounds					

#20 ENDURANCE

WORKOUT

T-Push Ups, Sandbag Step Ups, Sandbag Goblet Squats, Sandbag Clean & Press, Pull Ups.

Perform each exercise for 1 minute, giving a total round of 5 minutes. Record the number of repetitions performed within each minute for each exercise. There is a 1 minute rest period between each set of 5 exercises but a running clock during each round. Repeat for 3 rounds in total.

MEASUREMENT

Record your total repetitions for the whole sequence. Record the weight of the sandbag you used to complete this workout.

TARGET WEIGHT

Aim for a sandbag weighing 40% of your body weight

Date					
Reps/ Weight/ Time/ Rounds					

PART 4
POWER WORKOUTS

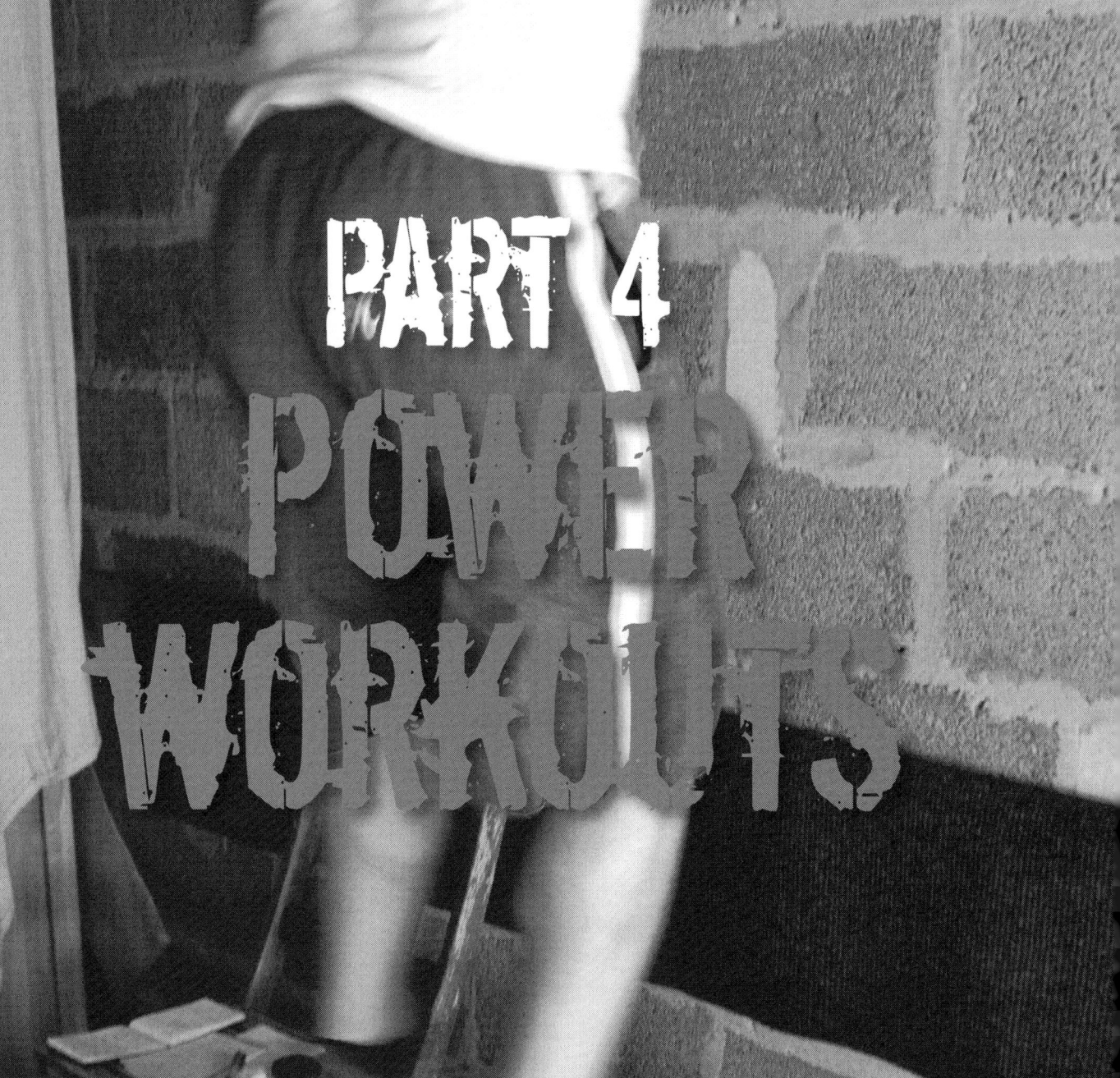

Power

verb | pow·er

1. To move with great speed or force.

Use these workouts to build, develop and maintain your physical power.

Power can be described as a combination of strength and speed, so you should aim to utilise both during these workouts. You'll typically find these workouts emphasising longer rest periods in order to keep the quality of the work high.

When working on your power the key is to fine tune the sandbag weight and the amount of speed you can generate with it. Too light a bag and you'll move into endurance territory; too heavy and it becomes a strength session. A moderate weight sandbag moved with as much speed as you can generate is a good rule of thumb.

POWER

"ALWAYS CHOOSE INTENSITY OVER VOLUME. WHEN IN DOUBT, DO LESS SETS OR LESS REPS, BUT GO HEAVIER. WHEN IN DOUBT, GO FASTER, NOT LONGER."

DAN JOHN

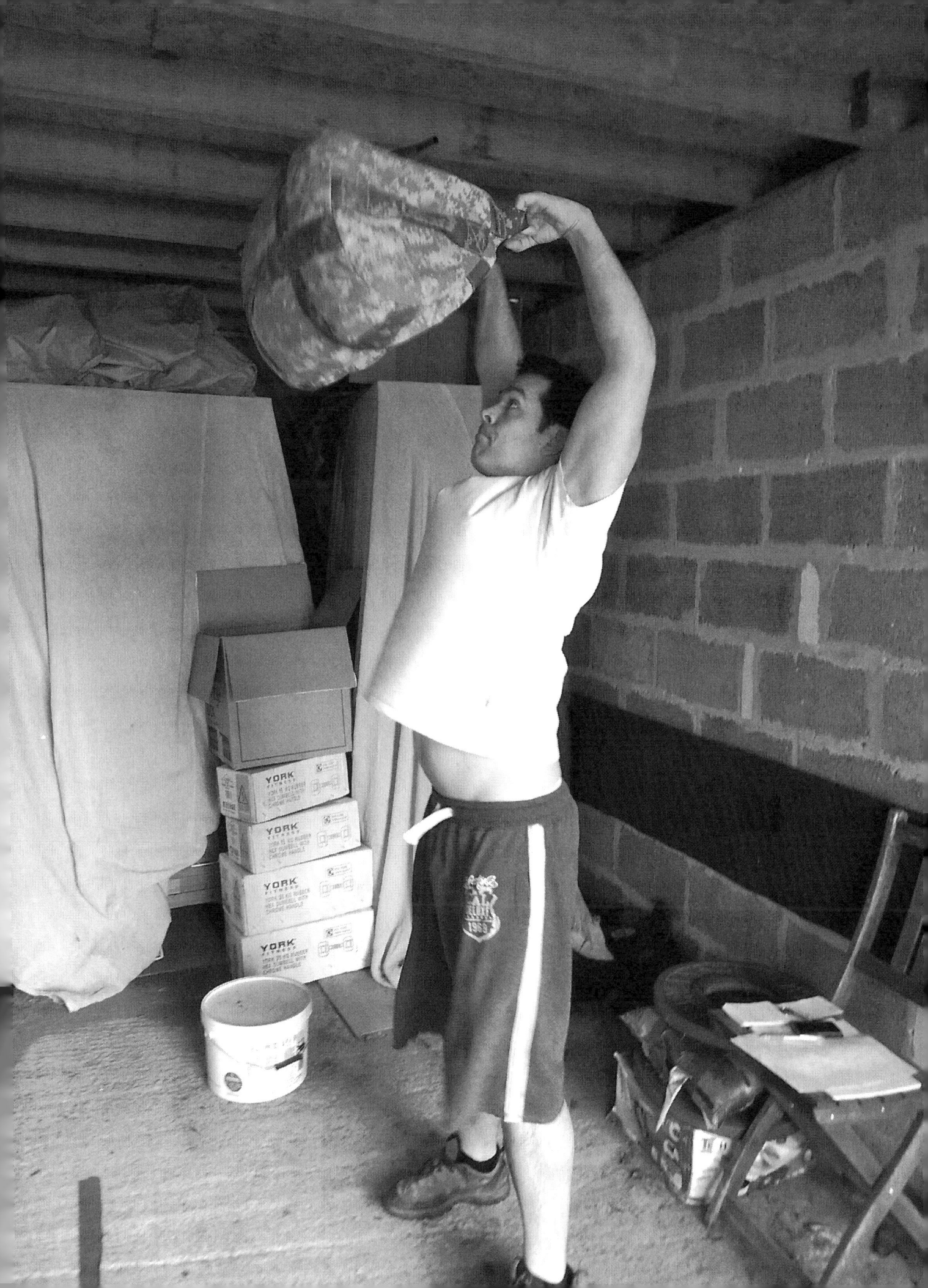

#1 POWER

WORKOUT

20 Sandbag Swings
10 Sandbag Snatches

Rest for 1 minute between rounds and repeat for a total of 5 rounds.

MEASUREMENT

Aim to complete the workout in as fast a time as you can. Record the weight of the sandbag you used to complete this workout.

TARGET WEIGHT

Aim for a sandbag weighing 40% of your body weight

Date					
Reps/ Weight/ Time/ Rounds					

#2 POWER

WORKOUT

Sandbag Clean & Forward Throw
5 Burpees

Run to the bag and repeat for a total of 20 rounds.

MEASUREMENT

Aim to complete the workout in as fast a time as you can. Record the weight of the sandbag you used to complete this workout.

TARGET WEIGHT

Aim for a sandbag weighing 30% of your body weight

Date					
Reps/ Weight/ Time/ Rounds					

#3 POWER

WORKOUT

5 Sandbag Clean & Push Jerk

Rest for 1 minute between rounds and repeat for a total of 5 rounds.

MEASUREMENT

Aim to complete the workout in as fast a time as you can. Record the weight of the sandbag you used to complete this workout.

TARGET WEIGHT

Aim for a sandbag weighing 75% of your body weight

Date					
Reps/ Weight/ Time/ Rounds					

#4 POWER

WORKOUT

Sprint 200m
10 Sandbag Push Press
20 Sandbag Round-the-Worlds (10 in each direction)

Rest for 1 minute between rounds and repeat for a total of 5 rounds.

MEASUREMENT

Aim to complete the workout in as fast a time as you can. Record the weight of the sandbag you used to complete this workout.

TARGET WEIGHT

Aim for a sandbag weighing 40% of your body weight, 20% for the Sandbag Round-the-Worlds

Date					
Reps/ Weight/ Time/ Rounds					

#5 POWER

WORKOUT

20 seconds of work, 10 seconds of rest - repeat for a total of 8 working intervals. 1 minute rest between exercises.

Sandbag High Pulls
Sandbag Round-the-Worlds (alternate sides between rounds)
Sandbag Push Jerks

MEASUREMENT

Record your total repetitions for each exercise. Record the weight of the sandbag you used to complete this workout.

TARGET WEIGHT

Aim for a sandbag weighing 40% of your body weight, 20% for the Round-the-Worlds

Date					
Reps/ Weight/ Time/ Rounds					

#6 POWER

WORKOUT

10 Sandbag Jump Squats
20 Sandbag High Pulls

Rest for 30 seconds between rounds and repeat for a total of 10 rounds.

MEASUREMENT

Aim to complete the workout in as fast a time as you can. Record the weight of the sandbag you used to complete this workout.

TARGET WEIGHT

Aim for a sandbag weighing 30% of your body weight

Date					
Reps/ Weight/ Time/ Rounds					

#7 POWER

WORKOUT

10 Sandbag Snatch
10 Sandbag Clean & Forward Throw

Rest for 30 seconds between rounds and repeat for a total of 6 rounds.

MEASUREMENT

Aim to complete the workout in as fast a time as you can. Record the weight of the sandbag you used to complete this workout.

TARGET WEIGHT

Aim for a sandbag weighing 30% of your body weight

Date					
Reps/ Weight/ Time/ Rounds					

#8 POWER

WORKOUT

20 seconds of work, 10 seconds of rest - repeat for a total of 8 working intervals. 1 minute rest between exercises.

Box Jumps
Sandbag Thrusters
Sandbag High Pulls
Burpees

MEASUREMENT

Record your total repetitions for each exercise. Record the weight of the sandbag you used to complete this workout.

TARGET WEIGHT

Aim for a sandbag weighing 40% of your body weight

Date					
Reps/ Weight/ Time/ Rounds					

#9 POWER

WORKOUT

Sandbag Backwards Throw

Repeat for a total of 30 throws.

MEASUREMENT

Aim to cover the greatest distance in a total of 30 throws. Record the weight of the sandbag you used to complete this workout.

TARGET WEIGHT

Aim for a sandbag weighing 30% of your body weight

Date					
Reps/ Weight/ Time/ Rounds					

#10 POWER

WORKOUT

100m Sprint
20 Sandbag Swings
10 Sandbag Thrusters

Rest for 1 minute between rounds and repeat for a total of 5 rounds.

MEASUREMENT

Aim to complete the workout in as fast a time as you can. Record the weight of the sandbag you used to complete this workout.

TARGET WEIGHT

Aim for a sandbag weighing 30% of your body weight

Date					
Reps/ Weight/ Time/ Rounds					

PART 5
AGILITY WORKOUTS

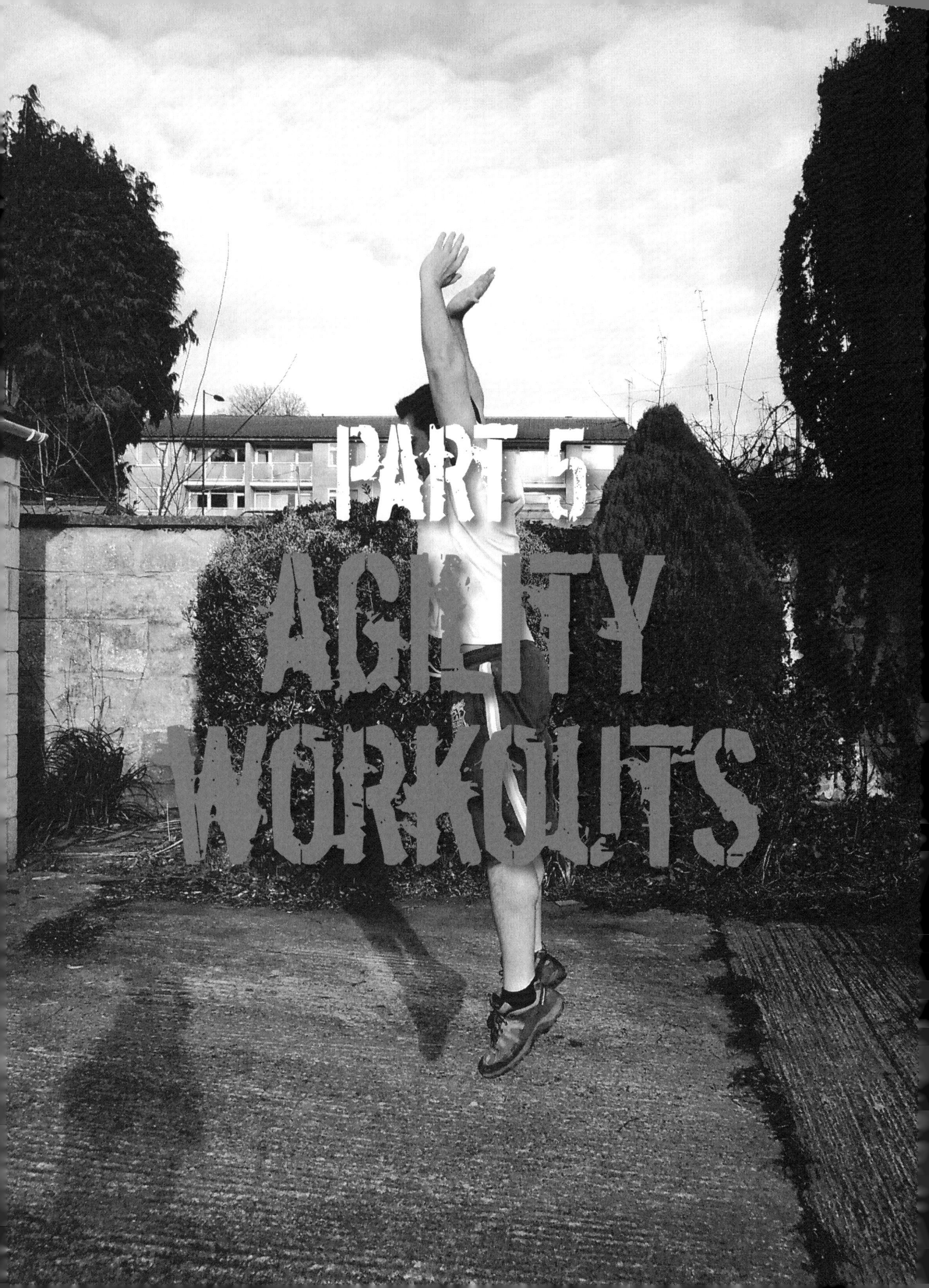

Agility

noun | agil·i·ty

1. The quality or state of being agile.

Use these workouts to build, develop and maintain your agility.

The workouts in this section are focused on multi-planar movement and stress.

When working on your agility the key is to stay loose and work to avoid any excessive fatigue. Being able to move freely, with good technique, becomes very challenging when fatigue sets it. Don't be afraid to utilise longer and more frequent rest periods in order to keep the quality of the work high.

AGILITY

> "THE ONE WHO DOESN'T FALL, DOESN'T STAND UP."
>
> — FEDOR EMELIANENKO

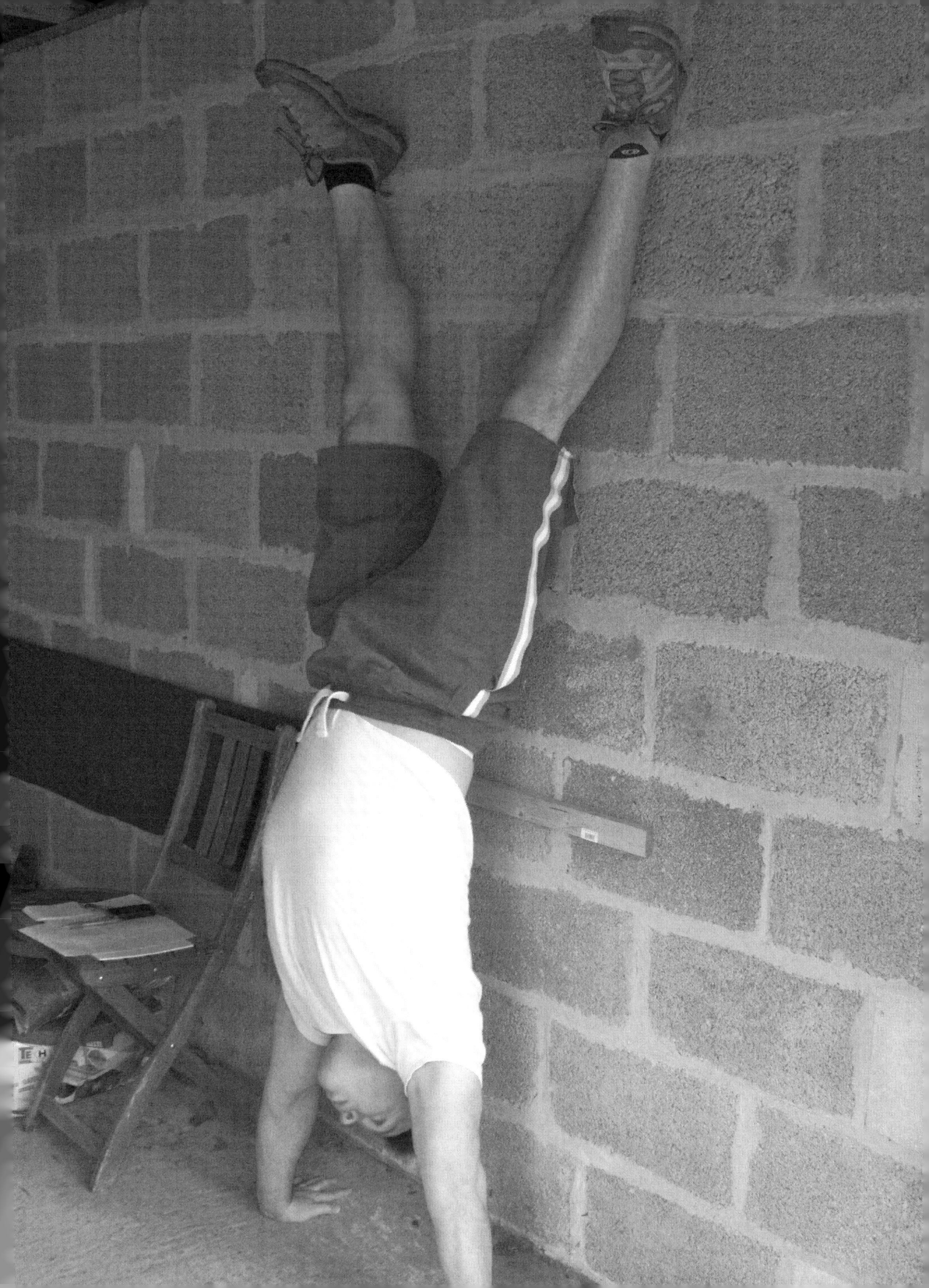

#1 AGILITY

WORKOUT

20 - 1 of the following exercises (perform 20 repetitions of each one, then 19 etc.):

Sandbag Thrusters
Burpees
Knees to Elbows

MEASUREMENT

Aim to complete the workout in as fast a time as you can. Record the weight of the sandbag you used to complete this workout.

TARGET WEIGHT

Aim for a sandbag weighing 30% of your body weight

Date					
Reps/ Weight/ Time/ Rounds					

#2 AGILITY

WORKOUT

10 Sandbag Bridge Floor Press
1 Sandbag Get Up (each side)
10 Shoulder-to-Shoulder Sandbag Press (5 each side)

As many rounds as possible in 5 minutes, rest for 1 minute and repeat for a total of 3 rounds.

MEASUREMENT

Record the number of rounds you can complete in each 5 minute period. Record the weight of the sandbag you used to complete this workout.

TARGET WEIGHT

Aim for a sandbag weighing 30% of your body weight

Date					
Reps/ Weight/ Time/ Rounds					

#3 AGILITY

WORKOUT

10 - 1 of the following exercises (perform 10 repetitions of each one, then 9 etc.):

Sandbag Clean & Press
Burpees
Handstand Push Ups

MEASUREMENT

Aim to complete the workout in as fast a time as you can. Record the weight of the sandbag you used to complete this workout.

TARGET WEIGHT

Aim for a sandbag weighing 30% of your body weight

Date					
Reps/ Weight/ Time/ Rounds					

#4 AGILITY

WORKOUT

20 Box Jumps
20 Sandbag Zercher Walking Lunges (10 each side)
20 Sandbag Round-the-Worlds (10 each side)

Repeat for a total of 8 rounds.

MEASUREMENT

Aim to complete the workout in as fast a time as you can. Record the weight of the sandbag you used to complete this workout.

TARGET WEIGHT

Aim for a sandbag weighing 30% of your body weight, 15% for the Round-the-Worlds

Date					
Reps/ Weight/ Time/ Rounds					

#5 AGILITY

WORKOUT

Sandbag Thruster Burpees

Every minute, on the minute. In minute 1 perform 1 repetition of the exercise, in minute 2 perform 2 repetitions of the exercise etc. Keep going until you can no longer complete the required repetitions.

MEASUREMENT

Record the number of rounds you can complete before reaching failure. Record the weight of the sandbag you used to complete this workout.

TARGET WEIGHT

Aim for a sandbag weighing 30% of your body weight

Date					
Reps/ Weight/ Time/ Rounds					

#6 AGILITY

WORKOUT

10 Sandbag Front Lateral Lunges (5 each side)
10 Sandbag Windmills (5 each side)
10 Sandbag Shoulder Get Ups (5 each side)

Repeat for a total of 5 rounds.

MEASUREMENT

Aim to complete the workout in as fast a time as you can. Record the weight of the sandbag you used to complete this workout.

TARGET WEIGHT

Aim for a sandbag weighing 30% of your body weight

Date					
Reps/ Weight/ Time/ Rounds					

#7 AGILITY

WORKOUT

20 Sandbag Step-Ups (10 each side)
10 Sandbag Jump Squats

Complete as many rounds as possible in 15 minutes.

MEASUREMENT

Record the number of rounds you can complete in 15 minutes. Record the weight of the sandbag you used to complete this workout.

TARGET WEIGHT

Aim for a sandbag weighing 30% of your body weight

Date					
Reps/ Weight/ Time/ Rounds					

#8 AGILITY

WORKOUT

20 Sandbag Overhead Lateral Lunges (10 each side)
10 Sandbag Bridge Floor Press
10 Sandbag Get Ups (5 each side)

Repeat for a total of 5 rounds.

MEASUREMENT

Aim to complete the workout in as fast a time as you can. Record the weight of the sandbag you used to complete this workout.

TARGET WEIGHT

Aim for a sandbag weighing 30% of your body weight

Date					
Reps/ Weight/ Time/ Rounds					

#9 AGILITY

WORKOUT

10 Burpees
15 Box Jumps
20m Sandbag Drag

Repeat for a total of 6 rounds.

MEASUREMENT

Aim to complete the workout in as fast a time as you can. Record the weight of the sandbag you used to complete this workout.

TARGET WEIGHT

Aim for a sandbag weighing 30% of your body weight

Date					
Reps/ Weight/ Time/ Rounds					

#10 AGILITY

WORKOUT

Sprint 50m
3 Sandbag Shoulder Get Ups (each side)
10 Sandbag Jump Squats

Repeat for a total of 5 rounds.

MEASUREMENT

Aim to complete the workout in as fast a time as you can. Record the weight of the sandbag you used to complete this workout.

TARGET WEIGHT

Aim for a sandbag weighing 30% of your body weight

Date					
Reps/ Weight/ Time/ Rounds					

PART 6
UPPER BODY WORKOUTS

Two tickets to the gun show.

Use these workouts to build, develop and maintain your upper body.

Where possible I always suggest balance in your workouts and a focus on the body as a whole. But balance doesn't always have to happen in each and every workout - that can sometimes lead to training sessions where you try too hard to fit everything in. When thinking about balancing the types of exercises, muscles used, and overall goal I prefer to look at my training over the course of 1-2 weeks. This allows you to get the most from each session without losing focus.

With that in mind, this section includes 10 Upper Body Workouts that are aimed at helping to develop Strength, Endurance, Agility and Power in the Arms, Shoulders, Chest and Back.

It should also be noted that the Upper Body workouts also place significant demands on the entire body.

UPPER BODY

> "IF THOSE GUYS WITH BETTER GENES TRAINED AS HARD AND INTENSE AS ME, I WOULDN'T STAND A CHANCE!"
>
> — DORIAN YATES

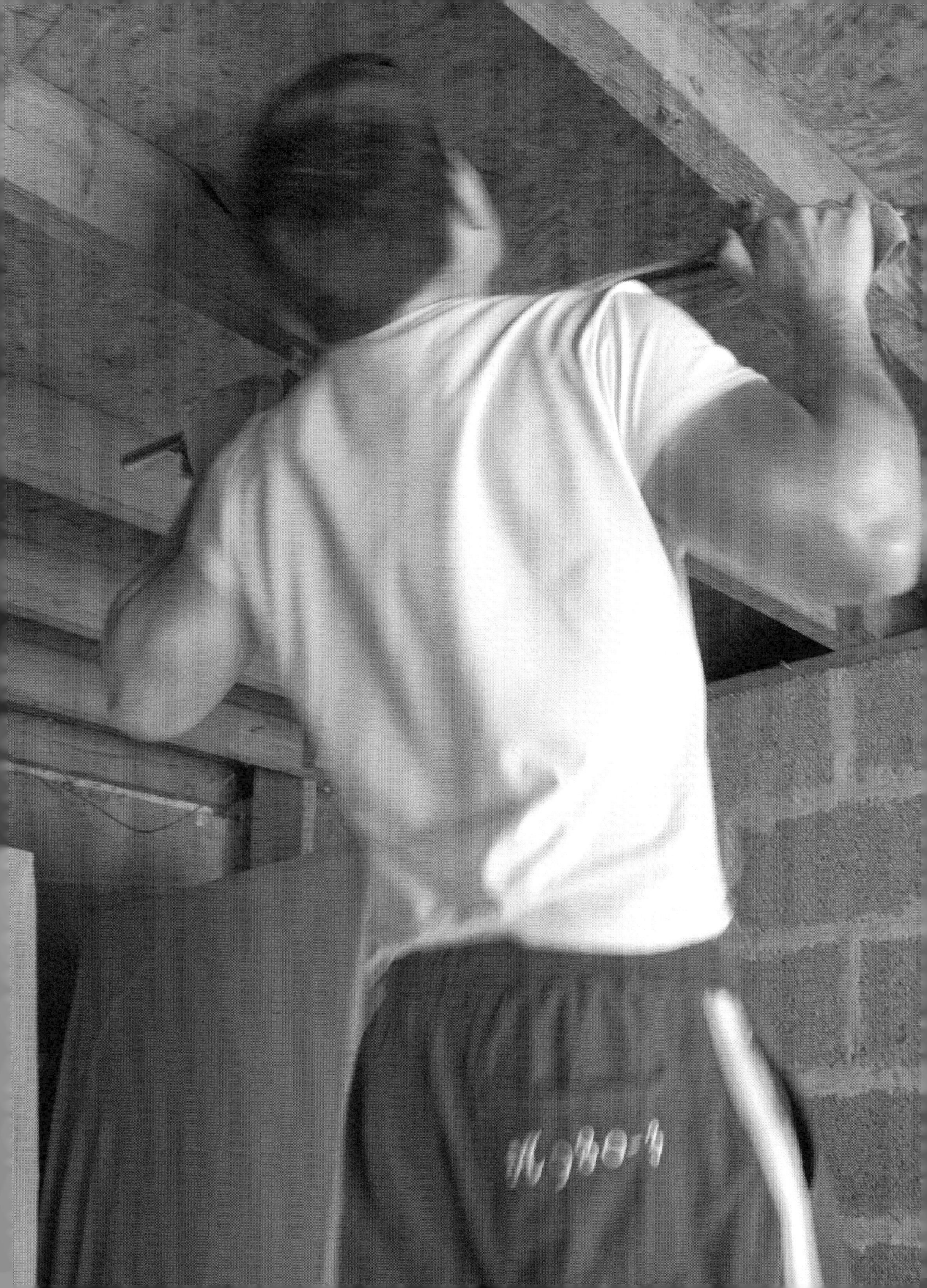

#1 UPPER BODY

WORKOUT

10 Sandbag Cleans
10 Sandbag Push Presses

Rest for 1 minute between rounds, and repeat for a total of 5 rounds.

MEASUREMENT

Aim to complete the workout in as fast a time as you can. Record the weight of the sandbag you used to complete this workout.

TARGET WEIGHT

Aim for a sandbag weighing 50% of your body weight

Date					
Reps/ Weight/ Time/ Rounds					

#2 UPPER BODY

WORKOUT

5 Pull Ups
10 Sandbag Upright Rows
15 Sandbag Push Press

Repeat for a total of 10 rounds.

MEASUREMENT

Aim to complete the workout in as fast a time as you can. Record the weight of the sandbag you used to complete this workout.

TARGET WEIGHT

Aim for a sandbag weighing 40% of your body weight

Date					
Reps/ Weight/ Time/ Rounds					

#3 UPPER BODY

WORKOUT

10 Sandbag Overhead Presses
10 Sandbag Bent-over-Rows
10 Sandbag Arm Curls

Rest for 1 minute between rounds, and repeat for a total of 5 rounds.

MEASUREMENT

Aim to complete the workout in as fast a time as you can. Record the weight of the sandbag you used to complete this workout.

TARGET WEIGHT

Aim for a sandbag weighing 50% of your body weight, 25% for the Arm Curls

Date					
Reps/ Weight/ Time/ Rounds					

#4 UPPER BODY

WORKOUT

Sandbag Push Jerks

Every minute, on the minute. In minute 1 perform 1 repetition of the exercise, in minute 2 perform 2 repetitions of the exercise etc. Keep going until you can no longer complete the required repetitions within that round.

MEASUREMENT

Record the number of rounds you can complete before reaching failure. Record the weight of the sandbag you used to complete this workout.

TARGET WEIGHT

Aim for a sandbag weighing 50% of your body weight

Date					
Reps/ Weight/ Time/ Rounds					

#5 UPPER BODY

WORKOUT

10 - 1 of the following exercises (perform 10 repetitions of each one, then 9 etc.):

Handstand Push Ups
Pull Ups
Sandbag Shoulder-to-Shoulder Press

MEASUREMENT

Aim to complete the workout in as fast a time as you can. Record the weight of the sandbag you used to complete this workout.

TARGET WEIGHT

Aim for a sandbag weighing 40% of your body weight

Date					
Reps/ Weight/ Time/ Rounds					

#6 UPPER BODY

WORKOUT

10 T-Push Ups
10 Sandbag Bent-over-Rows

Repeat for a total of 10 rounds.

MEASUREMENT

Aim to complete the workout in as fast a time as you can. Record the weight of the sandbag you used to complete this workout.

TARGET WEIGHT

Aim for a sandbag weighing 40% of your body weight

Date					
Reps/ Weight/ Time/ Rounds					

#7 UPPER BODY

WORKOUT

10 Sandbag High Pulls
10 Sandbag Floor Press
10 Sandbag Tricep Extensions

Rest for 1 minute between rounds, and repeat for a total of 5 rounds.

MEASUREMENT

Aim to complete the workout in as fast a time as you can. Record the weight of the sandbag you used to complete this workout.

TARGET WEIGHT

Aim for a sandbag weighing 50% of your body weight, 25% for the Tricep Extensions

Date					
Reps/ Weight/ Time/ Rounds					

#8 UPPER BODY

WORKOUT

Sandbag Bent-over-Rows
Sandbag Arm Curls

Every minute, on the minute. In minute 1 perform 1 repetition of each exercise, in minute 2 perform 2 repetitions of each exercise etc. Keep going until you can no longer complete the required repetitions.

MEASUREMENT

Record the number of rounds you can complete before reaching failure. Record the weight of the sandbag you used to complete this workout.

TARGET WEIGHT

Aim for a sandbag weighing 50% of your body weight, 25% for the Arm Curls

Date					
Reps/ Weight/ Time/ Rounds					

#9 UPPER BODY

WORKOUT

Sandbag Bent-over-Rows
Sandbag Overhead Press
Sandbag Arm Curls

Max repetitions in 5 minutes per exercise.

MEASUREMENT

Record the total number of repetitions you can complete in 15 minutes. Record the weight of the sandbag you used to complete this workout.

TARGET WEIGHT

Aim for a sandbag weighing 40% of your body weight, 20% for the Arm Curls

Date					
Reps/ Weight/ Time/ Rounds					

#10 UPPER BODY

WORKOUT

Sandbag Floor Press
Pull Ups

Every minute, on the minute. In minute 1 perform 1 repetition of each exercise, in minute 2 perform 2 repetitions of each exercise etc. Keep going until you can no longer complete the required repetitions.

MEASUREMENT

Record the number of rounds you can complete before reaching failure. Record the weight of the sandbag you used to complete this workout.

TARGET WEIGHT

Aim for a sandbag weighing 50% of your body weight

Date					
Reps/ Weight/ Time/ Rounds					

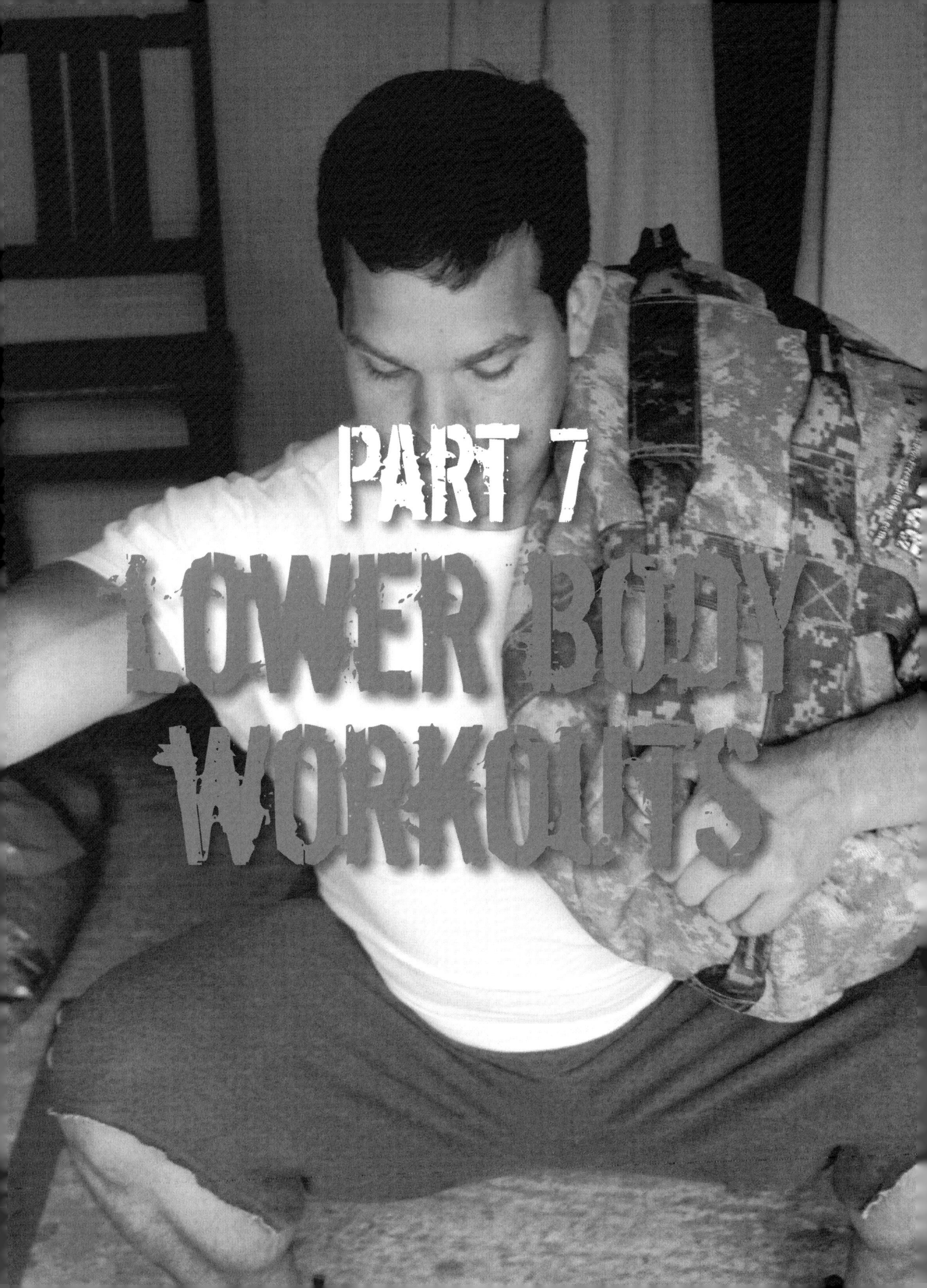

PART 7
LOWER BODY WORKOUTS

Part 7: Lower Body Workouts

Don't skip leg day.

Use these workouts to build, develop and maintain your lower body.

In much the same way that the Upper Body Workouts utilise other muscle groups, these Lower Body Workouts also place significant demands on the entire body.

With that in mind, this section includes 10 Lower Body Workouts that are aimed at helping to develop Strength, Endurance, Agility and Power in the Quads, Glutes, Hamstrings and Calves.

Part 7: Lower Body Workouts

LOWER BODY

> "THERE IS NEVER AN ABSOLUTE ANSWER TO EVERYTHING, EXCEPT OF COURSE THAT YOU HAVE TO DO YOUR SQUATS."
>
> — MARK RIPPETOE

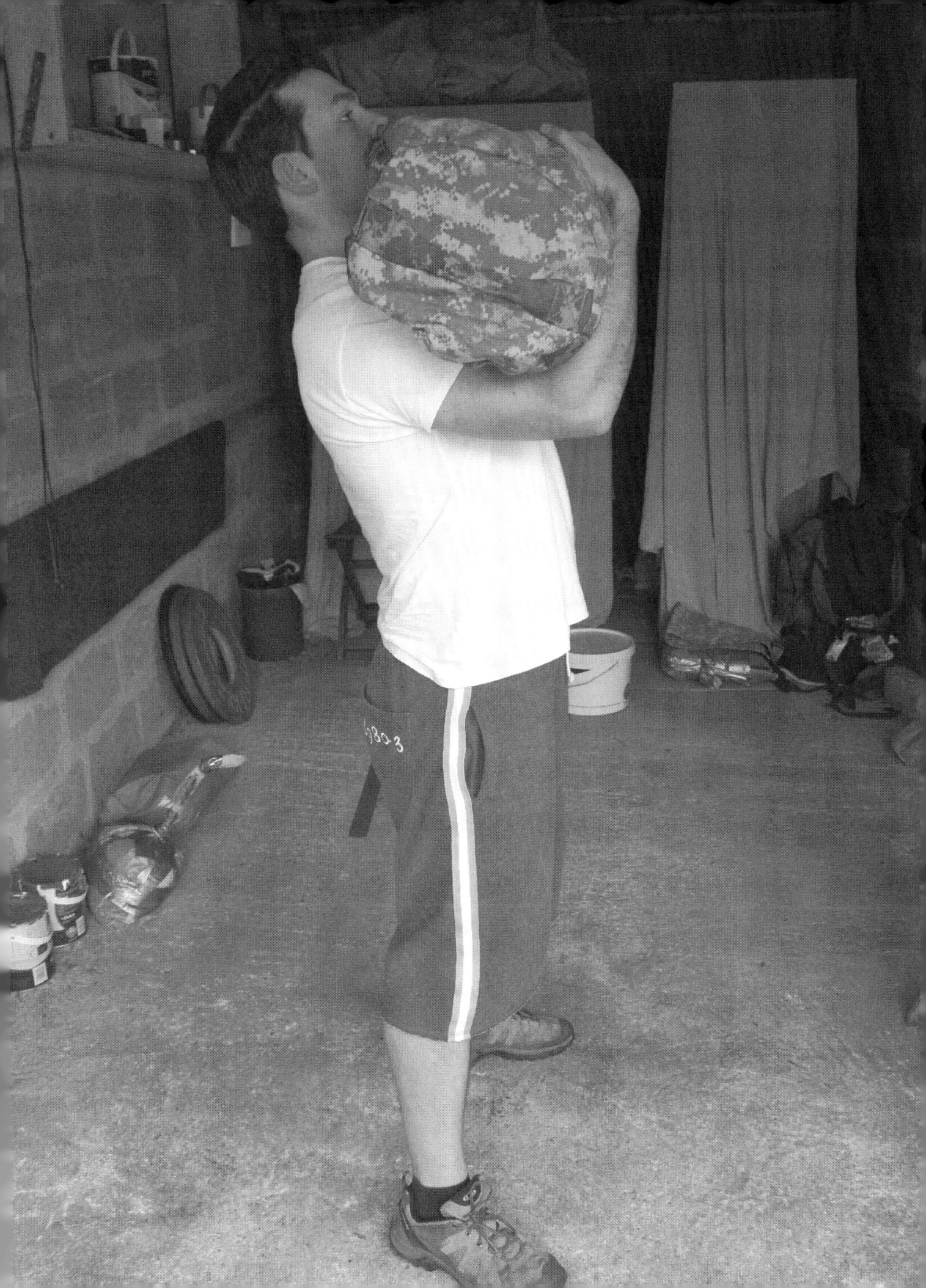

#1 LOWER BODY

WORKOUT

10 Sandbag Deadlifts
10 Sandbag Shoulder Squats
10 Sandbag Walking Lunges

Repeat for a total of 5 rounds.

MEASUREMENT

Aim to complete the workout in as fast a time as you can. Record the weight of the sandbag you used to complete this workout.

TARGET WEIGHT

Aim for a sandbag weighing 40% of your body weight

Date					
Reps/ Weight/ Time/ Rounds					

#2 LOWER BODY

WORKOUT

100m Sandbag Load Carry
100m Sandbag Drag

Repeat for a total of 5 rounds.

MEASUREMENT

Aim to complete the workout in as fast a time as you can. Record the weight of the sandbag you used to complete this workout.

TARGET WEIGHT

Aim for a sandbag weighing 60% of your body weight

Date					
Reps/ Weight/ Time/ Rounds					

Part 7: Lower Body Workouts

#3 LOWER BODY

WORKOUT

20 Sandbag Goblet Squats
20 Sandbag Hip Thrusts

Complete as many rounds as possible in 20 minutes.

MEASUREMENT

Record the number of rounds you can complete in 20 minutes. Record the weight of the sandbag you used to complete this workout.

TARGET WEIGHT

Aim for a sandbag weighing 50% of your body weight

Date					
Reps/ Weight/ Time/ Rounds					

#4 LOWER BODY

WORKOUT

5 Sandbag Bear Hug Squats
10 Sandbag Front Walking Lunges (5 each side)
20 Body weight Squats

Repeat for a total of 5 rounds.

MEASUREMENT

Aim to complete the workout in as fast a time as you can. Record the weight of the sandbag you used to complete this workout.

TARGET WEIGHT

Aim for a sandbag weighing 60% of your body weight

Date					
Reps/ Weight/ Time					

#5 LOWER BODY

WORKOUT

Sandbag Clean
Sandbag Zercher Squat

Every minute, on the minute. In minute 1 perform 1 repetition of each exercise, in minute 2 perform 2 repetitions of each exercise etc. Keep going until you can no longer complete the required repetitions within that round.

MEASUREMENT

Record the number of rounds you can complete before reaching failure. Record the weight of the sandbag you used to complete this workout.

TARGET WEIGHT

Aim for a sandbag weighing 40% of your body weight

Date					
Reps/ Weight/ Time/ Rounds					

#6 LOWER BODY

WORKOUT

200m Sandbag Load Carry
30 Body weight Squats

Repeat for a total of 5 rounds.

MEASUREMENT

Aim to complete the workout in as fast a time as you can. Record the weight of the sandbag you used to complete this workout.

TARGET WEIGHT

Aim for a sandbag weighing 50% of your body weight

Date					
Reps/ Weight/ Time/ Rounds					

#7 Lower Body

WORKOUT

10 Sandbag Split Squat (each side)
10 Sandbag Front Squats
10 Sandbag Calf Raises

Repeat for a total of 5 rounds.

MEASUREMENT

Aim to complete the workout in as fast a time as you can. Record the weight of the sandbag you used to complete this workout.

TARGET WEIGHT

Aim for a sandbag weighing 50% of your body weight

Date					
Reps/ Weight/ Time/ Rounds					

#8 LOWER BODY

WORKOUT

20 Sandbag Hip Thrusts
10 Sandbag Front Squat

Rest for 1 minute between rounds, and repeat for a total of 5 rounds.

MEASUREMENT

Aim to complete the workout in as fast a time as you can. Record the weight of the sandbag you used to complete this workout.

TARGET WEIGHT

Aim for a sandbag weighing 60% of your body weight

Date					
Reps/ Weight/ Time/ Rounds					

#9 LOWER BODY

WORKOUT

200 Skips
20 Sandbag Hip Thrusts
20 Box Jumps

Repeat for a total of 5 rounds.

MEASUREMENT

Aim to complete the workout in as fast a time as you can. Record the weight of the sandbag you used to complete this workout.

TARGET WEIGHT

Aim for a sandbag weighing 30% of your body weight

Date					
Reps/ Weight/ Time/ Rounds					

#10 LOWER BODY

WORKOUT

100m Sandbag Load Carry
30 Sandbag Step Ups (15 each side)
20 Sandbag Walking Lunges (10 each side)

Repeat for a total of 5 rounds.

MEASUREMENT

Aim to complete the workout in as fast a time as you can. Record the weight of the sandbag you used to complete this workout.

TARGET WEIGHT

Aim for a sandbag weighing 40% of your body weight

Date					
Reps/ Weight/ Time/ Rounds					

PART 8
SIMPLE WORKOUTS

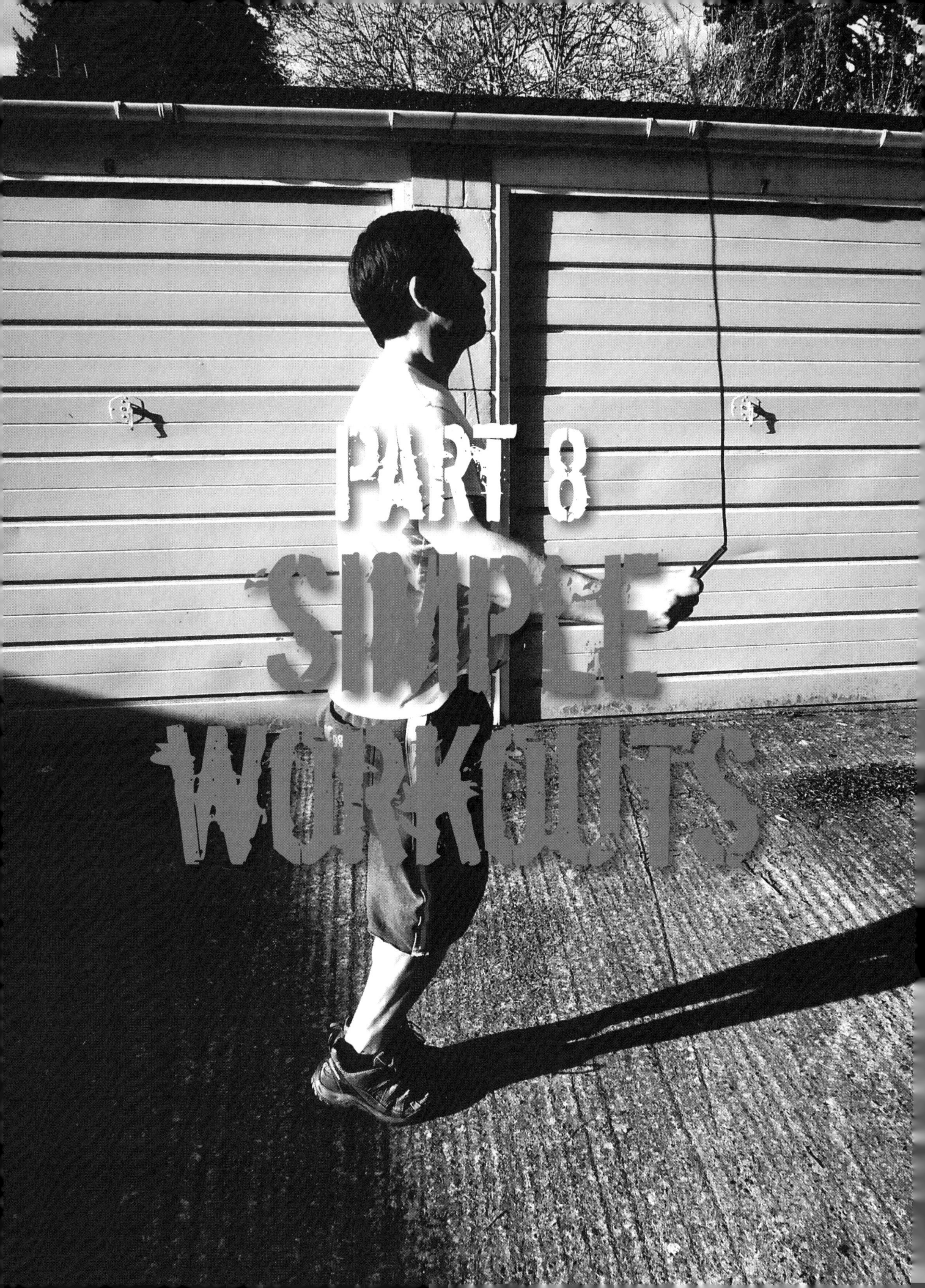

Simple

adjective | sim·ple | \sim-pel\

1. Not hard to understand or do.
2. Having few parts; not complex or fancy.
3. Not special or unusual.

The following workouts are designed to be simple to complete. That's not to say they aren't challenging, because they are, but they typically include a small number of individual exercises and those exercises aren't overly technical. As such it makes these workouts well suited to straightforward hard work.

The workouts detailed in this section also allow you to focus on the basics. Once you are able to master the basics, everything gets better.

114 Part 8: Simple Workouts

SIMPLE

"IT'S NOT THE DAILY INCREASE BUT THE DAILY DECREASE. HACK AWAY AT THE UNESSENTIAL."

BRUCE LEE

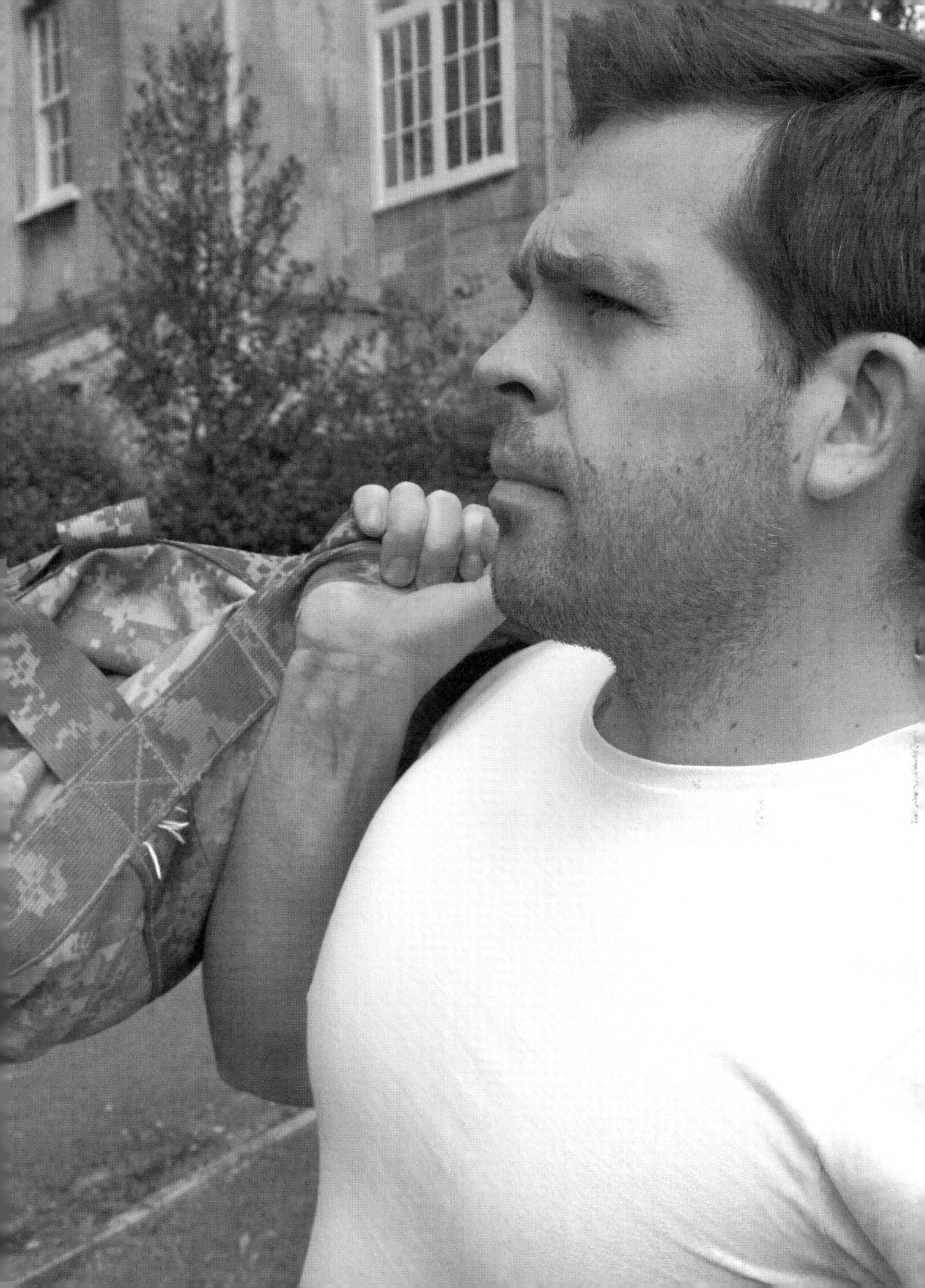

#1 SIMPLE

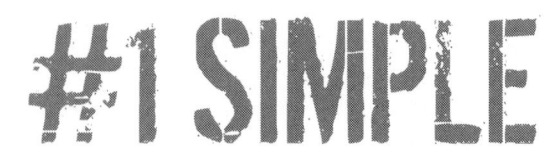

WORKOUT

100 Skips
20 Sandbag Thrusters

Repeat for a total of 5 rounds.

MEASUREMENT

Aim to complete the workout in as fast a time as you can. Record the weight of the sandbag you used to complete this workout.

TARGET WEIGHT

Aim for a sandbag weighing 50% of your body weight

Date					
Reps/ Weight/ Time/ Rounds					

#2 SIMPLE

WORKOUT

100 Sandbag Shoulders (50 each side)

MEASUREMENT

Aim to complete the workout in as fast a time as you can. Record the weight of the sandbag you used to complete this workout.

TARGET WEIGHT

Aim for a sandbag weighing 50% of your body weight

Date					
Reps/ Weight/ Time/ Rounds					

#3 SIMPLE

WORKOUT

5 Pull Ups
10 Sandbag Thrusters

Repeat for a total of 10 rounds.

MEASUREMENT

Aim to complete the workout in as fast a time as you can. Record the weight of the sandbag you used to complete this workout.

TARGET WEIGHT

Aim for a sandbag weighing 40% of your body weight

Date					
Reps/ Weight/ Time/ Rounds					

#4 SIMPLE

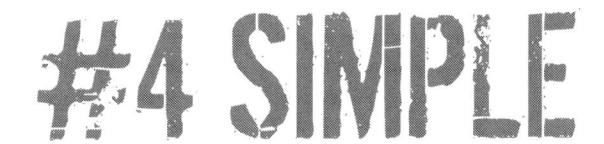

WORKOUT

10 Sandbag Zercher Squats
5 Sandbag Shoulder Get-Ups (switch shoulders each round)

Complete as many rounds as possible in 20 minutes.

MEASUREMENT

Record the number of rounds you can complete in 20 minutes. Record the weight of the sandbag you used to complete this workout.

TARGET WEIGHT

Aim for a sandbag weighing 40% of your body weight

Date					
Reps/ Weight/ Time/ Rounds					

Part 8: Simple Workouts

#5 SIMPLE

WORKOUT

10 Push Ups
15 Sandbag Deadlifts

Repeat for a total of 10 rounds.

MEASUREMENT

Aim to complete the workout in as fast a time as you can. Record the weight of the sandbag you used to complete this workout.

TARGET WEIGHT

Aim for a sandbag weighing 75% of your body weight

Date					
Reps/ Weight/ Time/ Rounds					

#6 SIMPLE

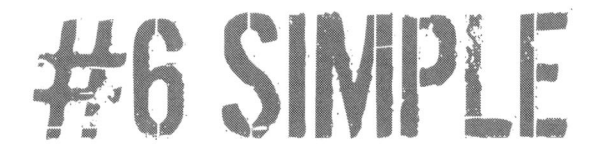

WORKOUT

Sandbag Floor Press
Sandbag Bear Hug Squat

Every minute, on the minute. In minute 1 perform 1 repetition of each exercise, in minute 2 perform 2 repetitions of each exercise etc. Keep going until you can no longer complete the required repetitions.

MEASUREMENT

Record the number of rounds you can complete before reaching failure. Record the weight of the sandbag you used to complete this workout.

TARGET WEIGHT

Aim for a sandbag weighing 30% of your body weight

Date					
Reps/ Weight/ Time/ Rounds					

#7 SIMPLE

WORKOUT

100 Sandbag Overhead Presses. You take a 100 Skip penalty every time you need to rest.

MEASUREMENT

Aim to complete the workout in as fast a time as you can. Record the weight of the sandbag you used to complete this workout.

TARGET WEIGHT

Aim for a sandbag weighing 40% of your body weight

Date					
Reps/ Weight/ Time/ Rounds					

#8 SIMPLE

WORKOUT

100m Sandbag Load Carry
10 Sandbag Clean & Press

Complete as many rounds as possible in 15 minutes.

MEASUREMENT

Record the number of rounds you can complete in 15 minutes. Record the weight of the sandbag you used to complete this workout.

TARGET WEIGHT

Aim for a sandbag weighing 30% of your body weight

Date					
Reps/ Weight/ Time/ Rounds					

#9 SIMPLE

WORKOUT

100 Sandbag Front Squats. You take a 20 Push Up penalty every time you need to rest.

MEASUREMENT

Aim to complete the workout in as fast a time as you can. Record the weight of the sandbag you used to complete this workout.

TARGET WEIGHT

Aim for a sandbag weighing 60% of your body weight

Date					
Reps/ Weight/ Time/ Rounds					

#10 SIMPLE

WORKOUT

Sandbag Thrusters

Every minute, on the minute. In minute 1 perform 1 repetition of the exercise, in minute 2 perform 2 repetitions of the exercise etc. Keep going until you can no longer complete the required repetitions.

MEASUREMENT

Record the number of rounds you can complete before reaching failure. Record the weight of the sandbag you used to complete this workout.

TARGET WEIGHT

Aim for a sandbag weighing 50% of your body weight

Date					
Reps/ Weight/ Time/ Rounds					

#11 SIMPLE

WORKOUT

25 Sandbag Deadlifts
25 Sandbag Good Mornings

Repeat for a total of 3 rounds.

MEASUREMENT

Aim to complete the workout in as fast a time as you can. Record the weight of the sandbag you used to complete this workout.

TARGET WEIGHT

Aim for a sandbag weighing 50% of your body weight

Date					
Reps/ Weight/ Time/ Rounds					

#12 SIMPLE

WORKOUT

Sandbag Clean
Sandbag Overhead Press

Max repetitions in 6 minutes per exercise.

MEASUREMENT

Record the total number of repetitions you can complete in 12 minutes. Record the weight of the sandbag you used to complete this workout.

TARGET WEIGHT

Aim for a sandbag weighing 50% of your body weight

Date					
Reps/ Weight/ Time/ Rounds					

#13 SIMPLE

WORKOUT

100 Sandbag Floor Press. You take a 20 Jump Squat penalty every time you need to rest.

MEASUREMENT

Aim to complete the workout in as fast a time as you can. Record the weight of the sandbag you used to complete this workout.

TARGET WEIGHT

Aim for a sandbag weighing 50% of your body weight

Date					
Reps/ Weight/ Time/ Rounds					

#14 SIMPLE

WORKOUT

10 - 1 of the following exercises (perform 10 repetitions of each one, then 9 etc.):

Sandbag Cleans
Sandbag Floor Press

MEASUREMENT

Aim to complete the workout in as fast a time as you can. Record the weight of the sandbag you used to complete this workout.

TARGET WEIGHT

Aim for a sandbag weighing 40% of your body weight

Date					
Reps/ Weight/ Time/ Rounds					

#15 SIMPLE

WORKOUT

100 Sandbag Thrusters. You take a 5 Pull Up penalty every time you need to rest.

MEASUREMENT

Aim to complete the workout in as fast a time as you can. Record the weight of the sandbag you used to complete this workout.

TARGET WEIGHT

Aim for a sandbag weighing 50% of your body weight

Date					
Reps/ Weight/ Time/ Rounds					

#16 SIMPLE

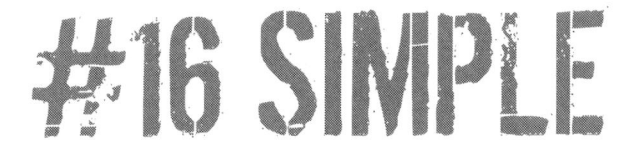

WORKOUT

200 Skips
20 Sandbag Swings

Repeat for a total of 5 rounds.

MEASUREMENT

Aim to complete the workout in as fast a time as you can. Record the weight of the sandbag you used to complete this workout.

TARGET WEIGHT

Aim for a sandbag weighing 30% of your body weight

Date					
Reps/ Weight/ Time/ Rounds					

#17 SIMPLE

WORKOUT

20 - 1 of the following exercises (perform 20 repetitions of each one, then 19 etc.):

Sandbag Back Squats (switch shoulders each round)
Knees-to-Elbows

MEASUREMENT

Aim to complete the workout in as fast a time as you can. Record the weight of the sandbag you used to complete this workout.

TARGET WEIGHT

Aim for a sandbag weighing 40% of your body weight

Date					
Reps/ Weight/ Time/ Rounds					

#18 SIMPLE

WORKOUT

Toes-to-Bar
Sandbag Upright Row

Every minute, on the minute. In minute 1 perform 1 repetition of the exercise, in minute 2 perform 2 repetitions of the exercise etc. Keep going until you can no longer complete the required repetitions.

MEASUREMENT

Record the number of rounds you can complete before reaching failure. Record the weight of the sandbag you used to complete this workout.

TARGET WEIGHT

Aim for a sandbag weighing 30% of your body weight

Date					
Reps/ Weight/ Time/ Rounds					

#19 SIMPLE

WORKOUT

20 T-Push Ups
20 Sandbag Back Squats

Repeat for a total of 5 rounds.

MEASUREMENT

Aim to complete the workout in as fast a time as you can. Record the weight of the sandbag you used to complete this workout.

TARGET WEIGHT

Aim for a sandbag weighing 50% of your body weight

Date					
Reps/ Weight/ Time/ Rounds					

#20 SIMPLE

WORKOUT

Sandbag Thrusters
Box Jumps

Max repetitions in 8 minutes per exercise.

MEASUREMENT

Record the total number of repetitions you can complete in 16 minutes. Record the weight of the sandbag you used to complete this workout.

TARGET WEIGHT

Aim for a sandbag weighing 40% of your body weight

Date					
Reps/ Weight/ Time/ Rounds					

PART 9
RUNNING WORKOUTS

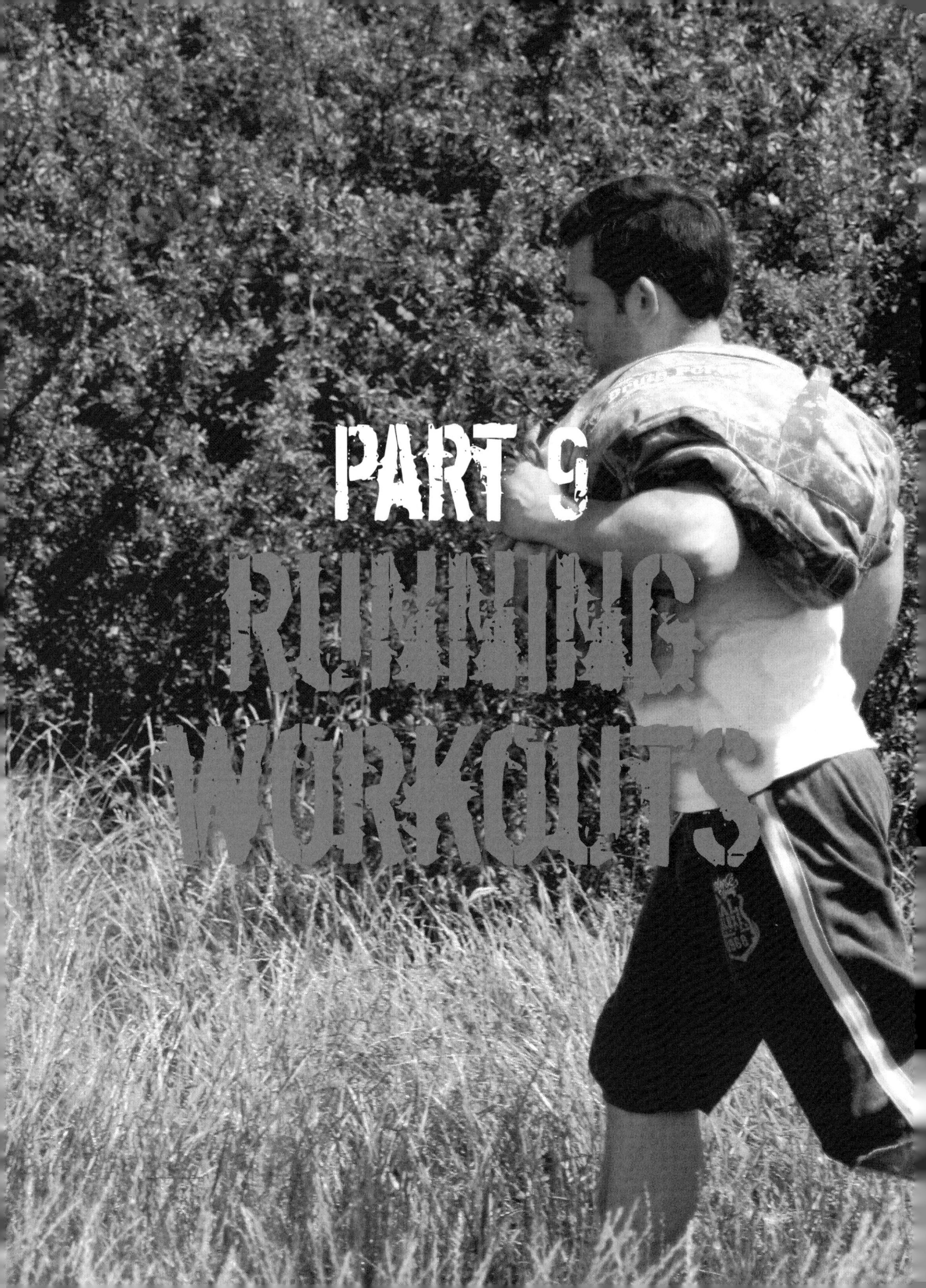

Running

noun | run·ning

1. The activity or sport of running.

Running has taken something of a bad rap in recent years. But a combination of sprinting, moderate distance running and lots of walking is a fantastic way to develop your athletic conditioning and improve general wellbeing.

In the following section the running distances are typically kept fairly short. This is done purposefully so that you are able to maintain a high intensity training session. Where possible any running you perform during these sessions should be fast.

138 Part 9: Running Workouts

RUNNING

"ONE THING ABOUT RACING IS THAT IT HURTS. YOU BETTER ACCEPT THAT FROM THE BEGINNING OR YOU'RE NOT GOING ANYWHERE."

BOB KENNEDY

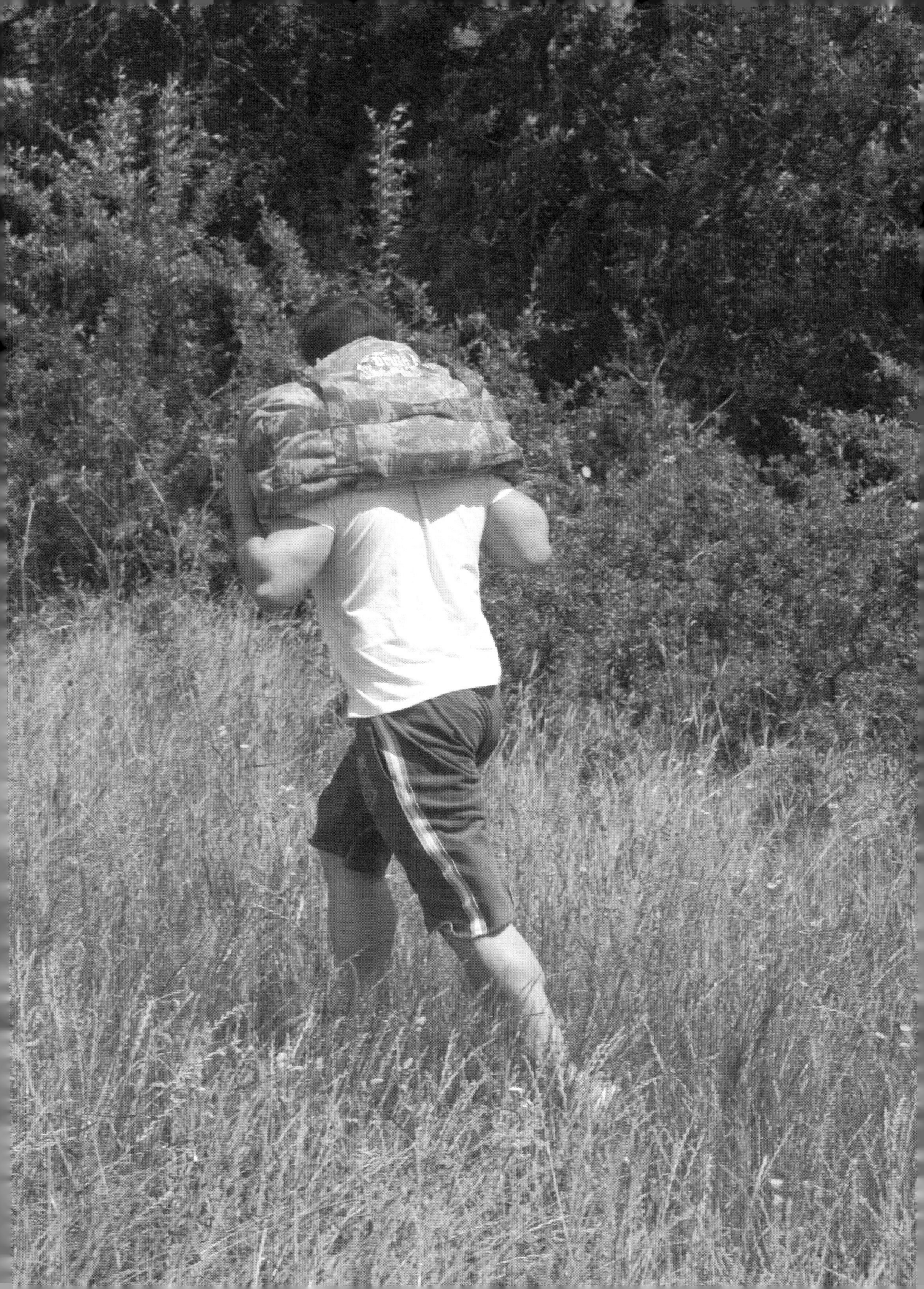

#1 RUNNING

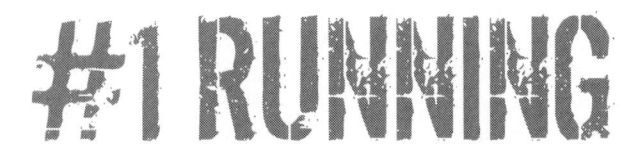

WORKOUT

Sprint 100m
20 Sandbag Floor Press
10 Sandbag Shoulder Get Ups (5 each side)

Complete as many rounds as you can in 15 minutes.

MEASUREMENT

Record the total number of rounds you can complete in 15 minutes. Record the sandbag weight used for the workout.

TARGET WEIGHT

Aim for a sandbag weighing 40% of your body weight

Date					
Reps/ Weight/ Time/ Rounds					

#2 RUNNING

WORKOUT

Run 1km
20 Sandbag Zercher Squats
20 Sandbag Push Press
20 Sandbag Shoulder Squats
20 Sandbag Bent-over-Rows
20 Sandbag Back Squats
Run 1km

MEASUREMENT

Aim to complete the workout in as fast a time as you can. Record the sandbag weight used for the workout.

TARGET WEIGHT

Aim for a sandbag weighing 40% of your body weight

Date					
Reps/ Weight/ Time/ Rounds					

#3 RUNNING

WORKOUT

Sprint 200m
5 Sandbag High Pulls
5 Sandbag Overhead Press
5 Sandbag Back Squats

Repeat for a total of 5 rounds.

MEASUREMENT

Aim to complete the workout in as fast a time as you can. Record the sandbag weight used for the workout.

TARGET WEIGHT

Aim for a sandbag weighing 50% of your body weight

Date					
Reps/ Weight/ Time/ Rounds					

#4 RUNNING

WORKOUT

50m Sandbag Hill Sprint (hold the sandbag as you wish)

Drag the sandbag back to the start and repeat for a total of 10 sprints.

MEASUREMENT

Aim to complete the workout in as fast a time as you can. Record the sandbag weight used for the workout.

TARGET WEIGHT

Aim for a sandbag weighing 40% of your body weight

Date					
Reps/ Weight/ Time/ Rounds					

#5 RUNNING

WORKOUT

Run 800m
21 Sandbag Thrusters
42 Box Jumps

Repeat for a total of 5 rounds as fast as you can.

MEASUREMENT

Aim to complete the workout in as fast a time as you can. Record the sandbag weight used for the workout.

TARGET WEIGHT

Aim for a sandbag weighing 30% of your body weight

Date					
Reps/ Weight/ Time/ Rounds					

#6 RUNNING

WORKOUT

Run 1km
25 Sandbag Clean & Press
25 Sandbag Shoulder Squats (each side)
Run 1km

MEASUREMENT

Aim to complete the workout in as fast a time as you can. Record the sandbag weight used for the workout.

TARGET WEIGHT

Aim for a sandbag weighing 50% of your body weight

Date					
Reps/ Weight/ Time/ Rounds					

#7 RUNNING

WORKOUT

Run 400m
20 Push Ups
30 Sit Ups
40 Sandbag Front Squats

Complete as many rounds as you can in 25 minutes.

MEASUREMENT

Record the total number of rounds you can complete in 25 minutes. Record the sandbag weight used for the workout.

TARGET WEIGHT

Aim for a sandbag weighing 30% of your body weight

Date					
Reps/ Weight/ Time/ Rounds					

#8 RUNNING

WORKOUT

Sprint 200m
20 Sandbag Floor Press
20 Sandbag Back Squats
20 Sandbag Round-the-Worlds (each side)

Repeat for a total of 5 rounds.

MEASUREMENT

Aim to complete the workout in as fast a time as you can. Record the sandbag weight used for the workout.

TARGET WEIGHT

Aim for a sandbag weighing 40% of your body weight, 20% for the Round-the-Worlds

Date					
Reps/ Weight/ Time/ Rounds					

#9 RUNNING

WORKOUT

Run 400m
10 Push Ups
20 Sandbag Cleans
30 Sandbag Back Squats

Repeat for a total of 5 rounds.

MEASUREMENT

Aim to complete the workout in as fast a time as you can. Record the sandbag weight used for the workout.

TARGET WEIGHT

Aim for a sandbag weighing 30% of your body weight

Date					
Reps/ Weight/ Time/ Rounds					

#10 RUNNING

WORKOUT

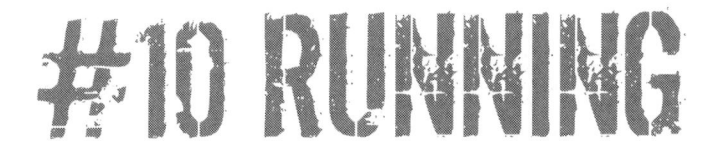

Sprint 200m
10 Push Ups
20 Sandbag Front Squats

Repeat for a total of 8 rounds.

MEASUREMENT

Aim to complete the workout in as fast a time as you can. Record the sandbag weight used for the workout.

TARGET WEIGHT

Aim for a sandbag weighing 40% of your body weight

Date					
Reps/ Weight/ Time/ Rounds					

PART 10
TEAM WORKOUTS

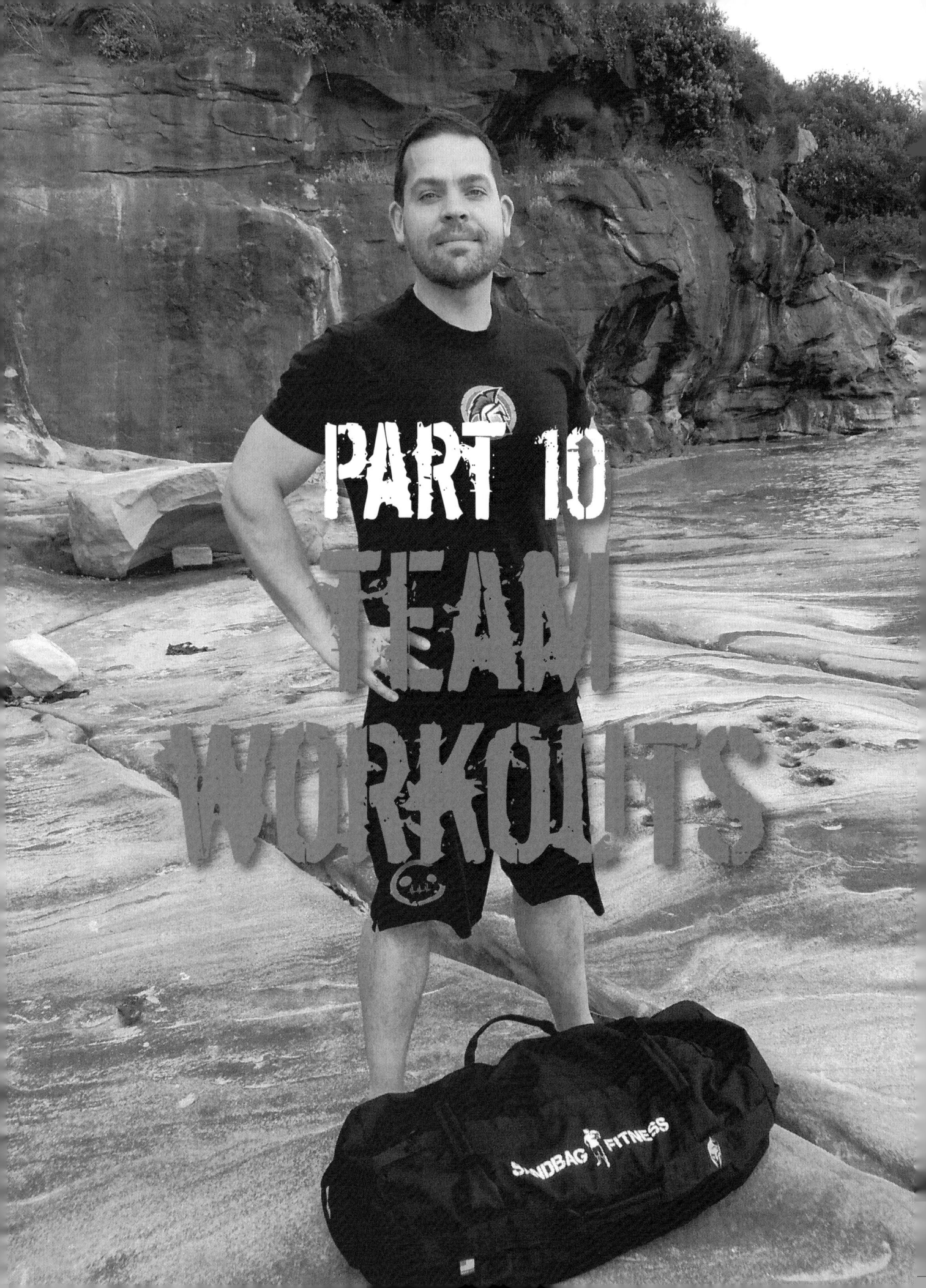

Team

noun | teem

1. A group of people who compete in a sport, game, etc., against another group.
2. A group of people who work together.

While training with a partner or as part of a team is certainly not vital to your success, in cannot be denied that if offers a whole different dimension to your fitness sessions. It's also fun! Where possible try to find training partners or a team that will challenge you - this will help to push your fitness even further.

The sessions detailed in this section can be used with a partner, a small group or as part of a large team, depending on your particular circumstances. In my experience the intensity of partner and small group sessions is always higher than that of large group sessions, where social loafing can occur. So, if you choose to train as part of a team then choose your training partners wisely.

TEAM WORKOUTS

"ONE MAN CAN BE A CRUCIAL INGREDIENT ON A TEAM, BUT ONE MAN CANNOT MAKE A TEAM."

KAREEM ABDUL-JABBAR

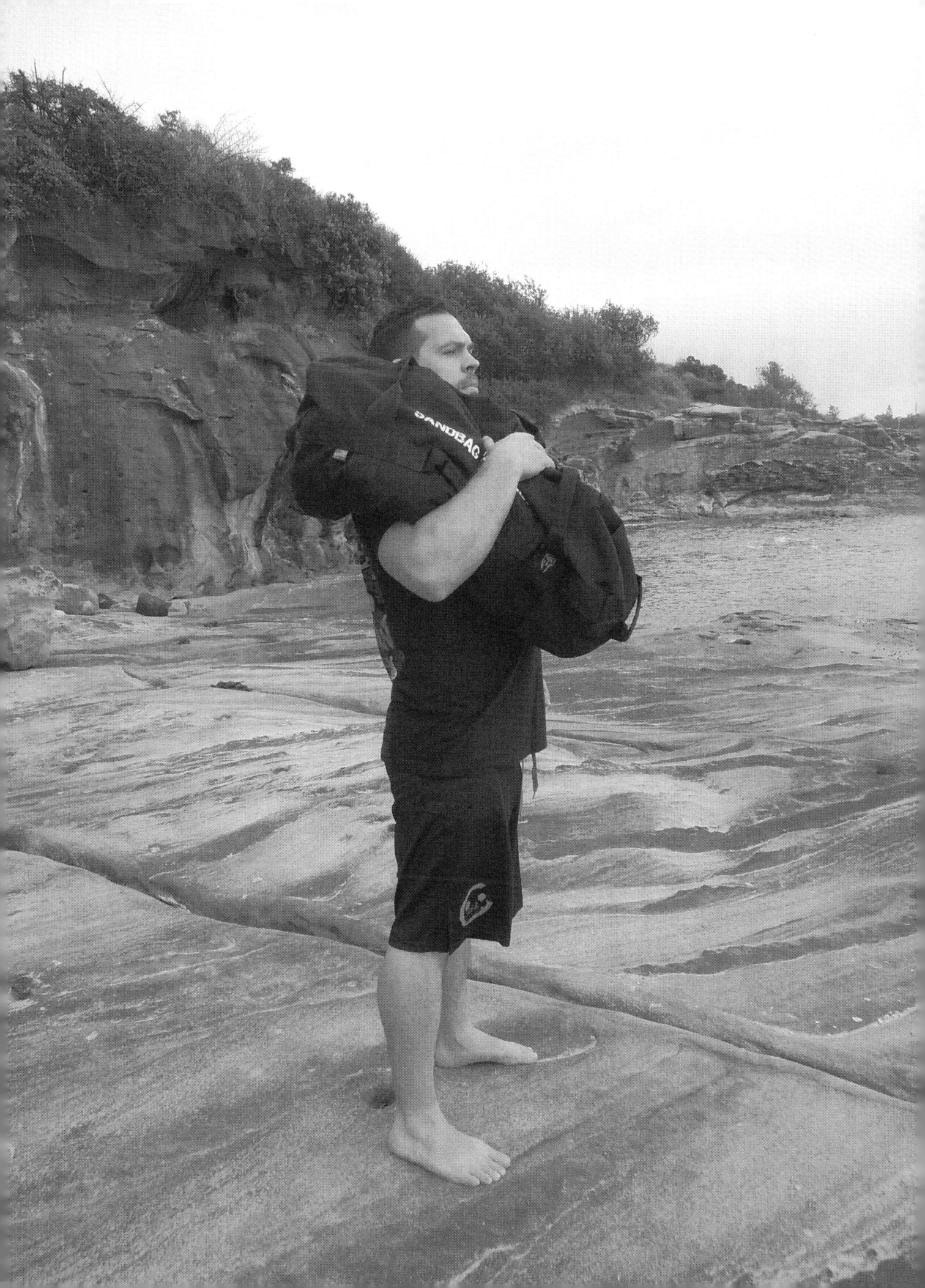

#1 TEAM

WORKOUT

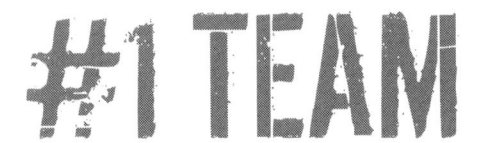

Sandball

Set out an area approximately 5m x 5m and designate a centre line (or put up a net). Divide into two teams. Start by chest passing the sandbag from one side of the court to the other. A member of the opposite team should chest catch it and then pass it back to the other side of the court again. Each time the sandbag drops to the ground the opposite team gets a point. If you're not using a net make sure you try to clear the imaginary net line with each pass.

MEASUREMENT

The first team or person to reach 20 points wins. Record the weight of the sandbag you used to complete this workout.

TARGET WEIGHT

Aim for a sandbag weighing 20% of the average body weight

Date					
Reps/ Weight/ Time/ Rounds					

#2 TEAM

WORKOUT

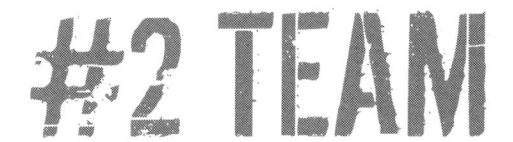

Sandbag Sumo

Set out an area approximately 5m x 5m. With a partner, take turns holding the sandbag at chest height while the opposing person tries to push you, via the sandbag, outside of the square. A point is scored each time the opposing player is pushed outside of the square or you manage to hold onto the sandbag for 1 minute, at which point you swap roles.

MEASUREMENT

The first person to reach 20 points wins. Record the weight of the sandbag you used to complete this workout.

TARGET WEIGHT

Aim for a sandbag weighing 40% of the average body weight

Date					
Reps/ Weight/ Time/ Rounds					

#3 TEAM

WORKOUT

Sandbag Catch

With a partner, stand facing each other, approximately 3m apart. Holding a sandbag at chest height, powerfully throw it to your partner. They catch the sandbag and pass it back to you.

Repeat for a total of 10 throws each. Rest for 1 minute and repeat for a total of 5 rounds.

MEASUREMENT

Aim to complete the workout in as fast a time as you can. Record the weight of the sandbag you used to complete this workout.

TARGET WEIGHT

Aim for a sandbag weighing 30% of the average body weight

Date					
Reps/ Weight/ Time/ Rounds					

#4 TEAM

WORKOUT

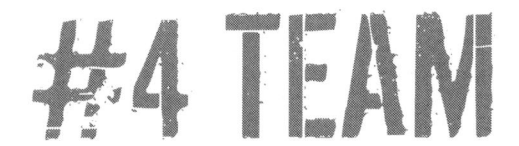

Sandbag Drag

Set out a course of 200m. Race to see who can drag their sandbag to the finish line the fastest.

MEASUREMENT

Aim to complete the workout in as fast a time as you can. Record the weight of the sandbag you used to complete this workout.

TARGET WEIGHT

Aim for a sandbag weighing 75% of the average body weight

Date					
Reps/ Weight/ Time/ Rounds					

#5 TEAM

WORKOUT

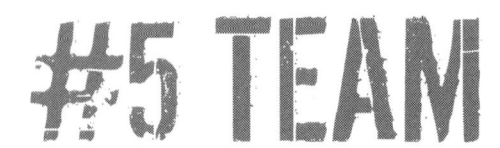

Sandbag Relay

Set out a course of approximately 20m. In pairs, perform a relay where each person takes it in turn to Sandbag Drag, Sandbag Load Carry and Sandbag Clean & Throw the sandbag along the course. This works best when performed with multiple pairs, all competing for time.

MEASUREMENT

The pair who complete the course in the fastest time are the winners. Record the weight of the sandbag you used to complete this workout.

TARGET WEIGHT

Aim for a sandbag weighing 50% of the average body weight

Date					
Reps/ Weight/ Time/ Rounds					

#6 TEAM

WORKOUT

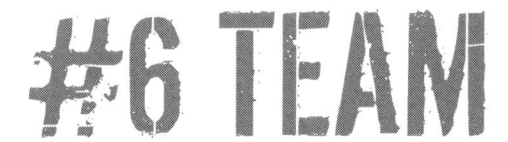

Sandbag Push 'n' Plank

In pairs, have 1 person adopt the Plank position while the other partner performs Sandbag Thrusters. Switch roles at the point of failure for either person.

Complete a total of 5 rounds each.

MEASUREMENT

Aim to complete as much time as possible. Record the weight of the sandbag you used to complete this workout.

TARGET WEIGHT

Aim for a sandbag weighing 30% of the average body weight

Date					
Reps/ Weight/ Time/ Rounds					

#7 TEAM

WORKOUT

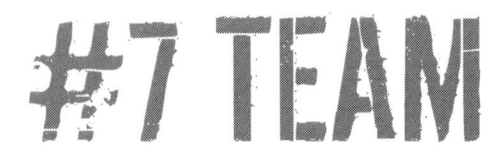

Sandbag Team Mile

Set out a course of 1 mile. With a partner, take it in turns to carry a sandbag any way you wish over the course.

MEASUREMENT

Aim to complete the workout in as fast a time as you can. Record the weight of the sandbag you used to complete this workout.

TARGET WEIGHT

Aim for a sandbag weighing 100% of the average body weight

Date					
Reps/ Weight/ Time/ Rounds					

#8 TEAM

WORKOUT

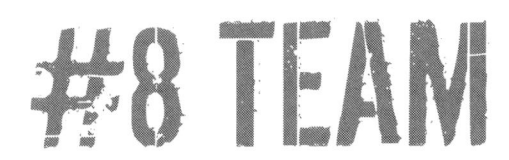

Sandbag Clean Off

With a partner, compete to see who can complete 50 Sandbag Clean & Press in the quickest time.

MEASUREMENT

Aim to complete the workout in as fast a time as you can. Record the weight of the sandbag you used to complete this workout.

TARGET WEIGHT

Aim for a sandbag weighing 50% of your body weight

Date					
Reps/ Weight/ Time/ Rounds					

#9 TEAM

WORKOUT

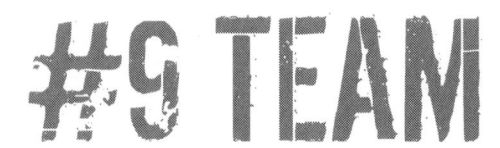

Sandbag Team Ladder

Sandbag Thrusters, Knees-to-Elbows

In a pair, go through the entire round performing just one of the exercises until either person reaches failure. At that stage switch exercises and perform again. In minute 1 perform 1 repetition of the exercise, in minute 2 perform 2 repetitions of the exercise etc.

MEASUREMENT

Aim to complete the workout in as fast a time as you can. Record the weight of the sandbag you used to complete this workout.

TARGET WEIGHT

Aim for a sandbag weighing 30% of the average body weight

Date					
Reps/ Weight/ Time/ Rounds					

#10 TEAM

WORKOUT

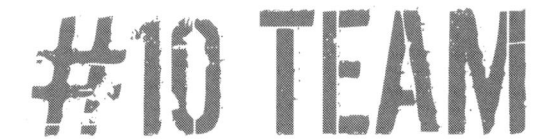

Sandbag Team Throw

Set out a course of approximately 50m. Everyone performs a Sandbag Clean & Forward Throw for maximum distance.

MEASUREMENT

The person who completes the 50m course with the fewest throws is the winner. Record the weight of the sandbag you used to complete this workout.

TARGET WEIGHT

Aim for a sandbag weighing 30% of your body weight

Date					
Reps/ Weight/ Time/ Rounds					

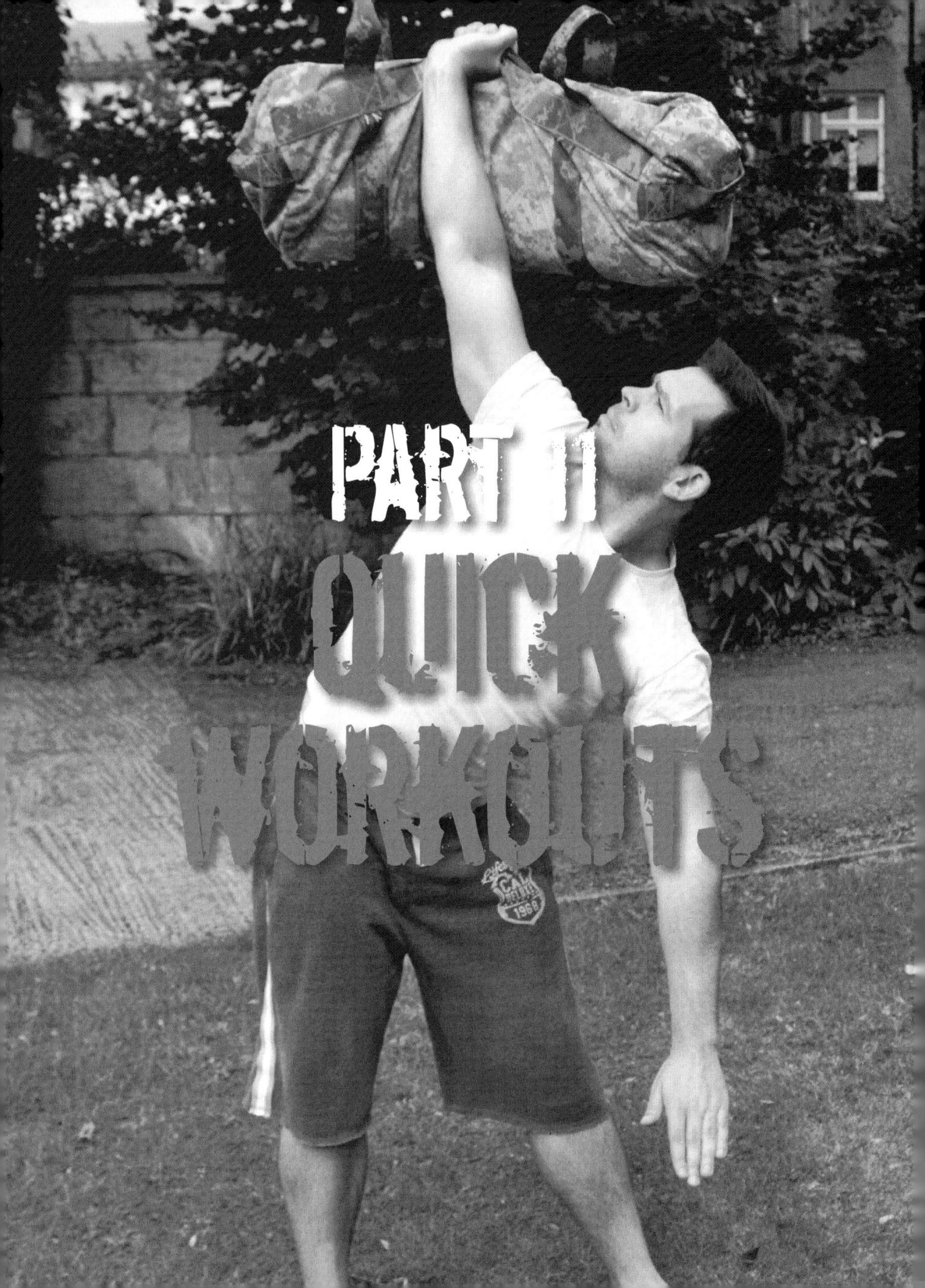

PART II
QUICK
WORKOUTS

Quick

adjective | \kwik\

1. Done or happening in a short amount of time.
2. Fast in thinking, learning, or understanding.
3. Fast in moving or reacting.

These workouts are designed to be completed in no more than 15 minutes, meaning that they are perfect for those times when you need to be quick. Even with a warm-up and cool-down you can be done in 30 minutes, with no excuses.

There are 20 Quick Workouts in total - ten 10 minute workouts, five 12 minute workouts, and five 15 minute workouts.

Quick is not a byword for rushed. Although you'll be focused on getting through the workout quickly, you should still maintain good technique.

QUICK

> "LIFE IS ABOUT TIMING."
> — CARL LEWIS

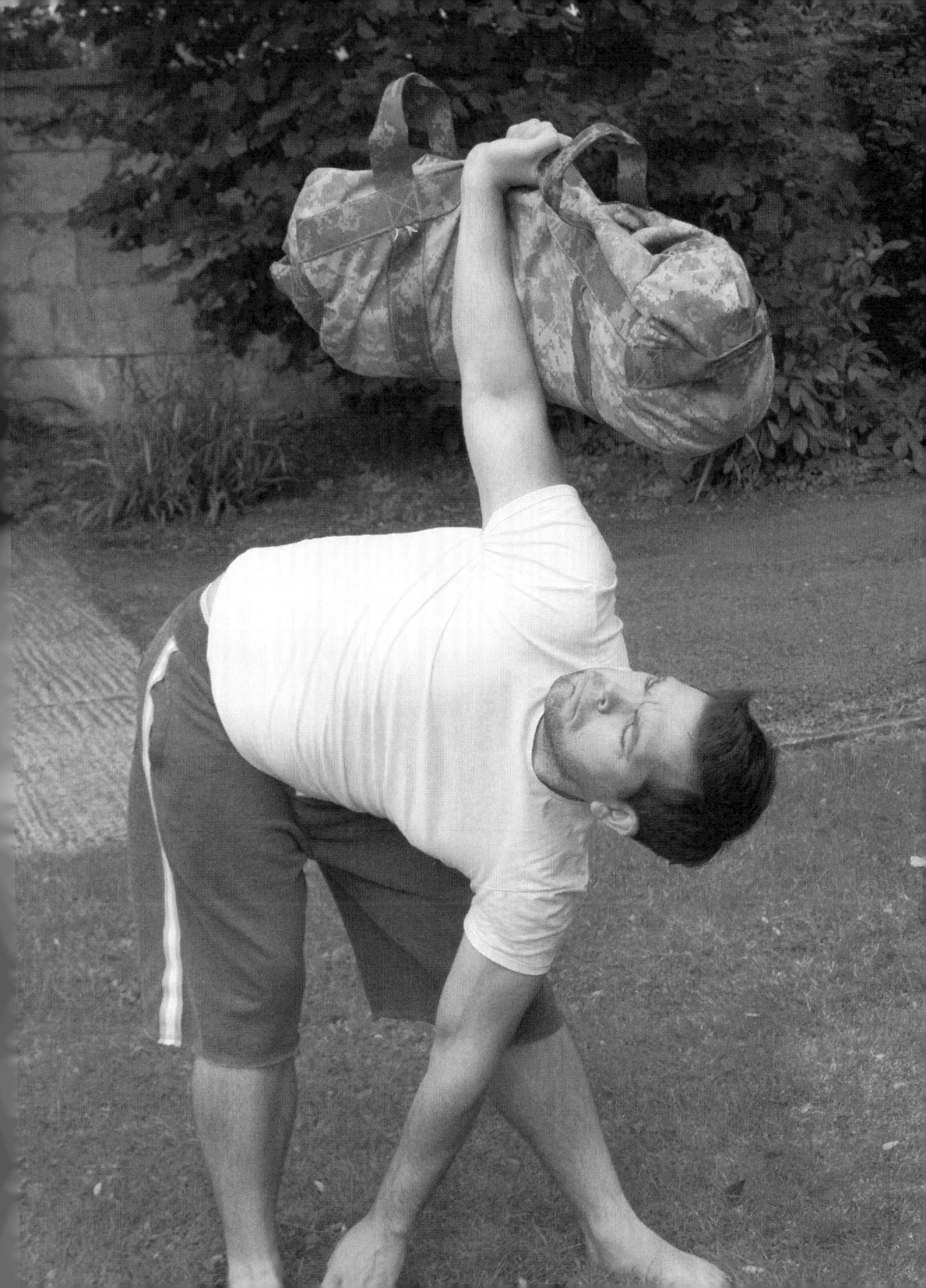

#1 QUICK

WORKOUT

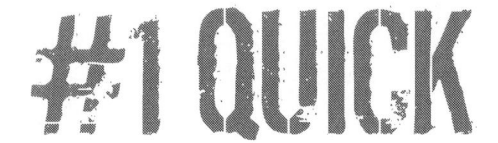

10 Sandbag Thrusters
5 Pull Ups

Aim to complete as many rounds as you can in 10 minutes.

MEASUREMENT

Record the total number of rounds you can complete in 10 minutes. Record the weight of the sandbag you used to complete this workout.

TARGET WEIGHT

Aim for a sandbag weighing 30% of your body weight

Date					
Reps/ Weight/ Time/ Rounds					

#2 QUICK

WORKOUT

Sandbag Shoulder Squats (switch shoulders as needed)
Sandbag Shoulder Get Ups (switch shoulders as needed)
Sandbag Cleans
Sandbag Push Press
Pull Ups

Max repetitions in 2 minutes per exercise.

MEASUREMENT

Record the total number of repetitions you can complete in 10 minutes. Record the weight of the sandbag you used to complete this workout.

TARGET WEIGHT

Aim for a sandbag weighing 30% of your body weight

Date					
Reps/ Weight/ Time/ Rounds					

#3 QUICK

WORKOUT

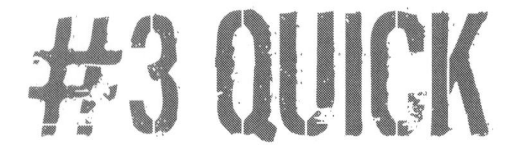

Sandbag Cleans
Sandbag Shouldering (switch sides each round)
Sandbag Good Mornings

Aim to complete as many rounds as you can in 10 minutes.

MEASUREMENT

Record the total number of rounds you can complete in 10 minutes. Record the weight of the sandbag you used to complete this workout.

TARGET WEIGHT

Aim for a sandbag weighing 30% of your body weight

Date					
Reps/ Weight/ Time/ Rounds					

#4 QUICK

WORKOUT

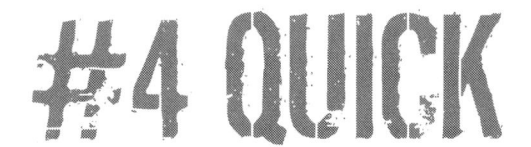

20 Sandbag Step Ups (10 each side)
10 Sandbag Get Ups (5 each side)

Aim to complete as many rounds as you can in 10 minutes.

MEASUREMENT

Record the total number of rounds you can complete in 10 minutes. Record the weight of the sandbag you used to complete this workout.

TARGET WEIGHT

Aim for a sandbag weighing 30% of your body weight

Date					
Reps/ Weight/ Time/ Rounds					

#5 QUICK

WORKOUT

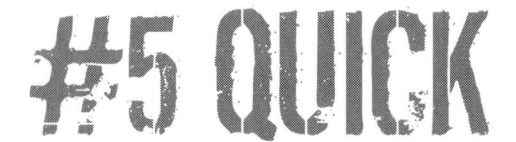

15 Sandbag High Pulls
15 Sandbag Cleans

Aim to complete as many rounds as you can in 10 minutes.

MEASUREMENT

Record the total number of rounds you can complete in 10 minutes. Record the weight of the sandbag you used to complete this workout.

TARGET WEIGHT

Aim for a sandbag weighing 30% of your body weight

Date					
Reps/ Weight/ Time/ Rounds					

#6 QUICK

WORKOUT

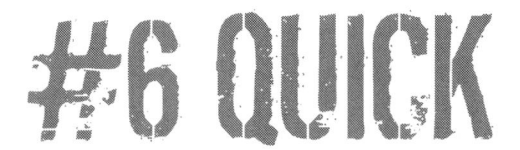

Sandbag Thrusters
Sandbag High Pulls

Max repetitions in 5 minutes per exercise.

MEASUREMENT

Record the total number of repetitions you can complete in 10 minutes. Record the weight of the sandbag you used to complete this workout.

TARGET WEIGHT

Aim for a sandbag weighing 40% of your body weight

Date					
Reps/ Weight/ Time/ Rounds					

#7 QUICK

WORKOUT

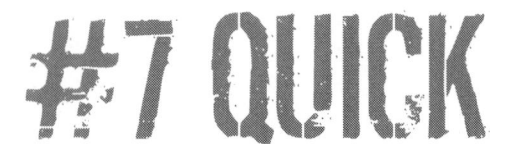

5 Sandbag Clean & Press
10 Sandbag Zercher Squats
15 Body weight Squats

Aim to complete as many rounds as you can in 10 minutes.

MEASUREMENT

Record the total number of rounds you can complete in 10 minutes. Record the weight of the sandbag you used to complete this workout.

TARGET WEIGHT

Aim for a sandbag weighing 30% of your body weight

Date					
Reps/ Weight/ Time/ Rounds					

#8 QUICK

WORKOUT

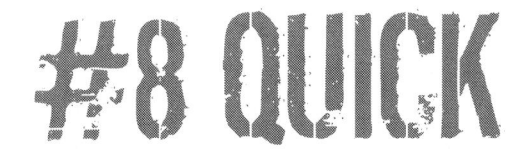

1 Sandbag Shoulder Get Up (each side)
5 Sandbag Thruster Burpees

Aim to complete as many rounds as you can in 10 minutes.

MEASUREMENT

Record the total number of rounds you can complete in 10 minutes. Record the weight of the sandbag you used to complete this workout.

TARGET WEIGHT

Aim for a sandbag weighing 30% of your body weight

Date					
Reps/ Weight/ Time/ Rounds					

#9 QUICK

WORKOUT

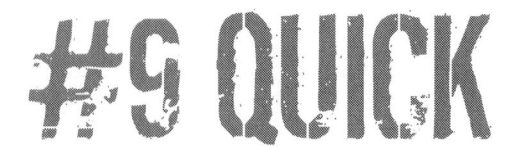

Sandbag Shoulder Get Ups (switch shoulders as needed)

Aim to complete as many repetitions as you can in 10 minutes.

MEASUREMENT

Record the total number of rounds you can complete in 10 minutes. Record the weight of the sandbag you used to complete this workout.

TARGET WEIGHT

Aim for a sandbag weighing 30% of your body weight

Date					
Reps/ Weight/ Time/ Rounds					

#10 QUICK

WORKOUT

Sandbag Thrusters, Sandbag Floor Press, Sandbag Bent-over-Row, Sandbag Good Mornings, Sandbag Swings.

Perform each exercise for 1 minute, giving a total round of 5 minutes. Record the number of repetitions performed within each minute for each exercise. Repeat for 2 rounds in total, with no rest between the rounds.

MEASUREMENT

Record your total repetitions for the whole sequence. Record the weight of the sandbag you used to complete this workout.

TARGET WEIGHT

Aim for a sandbag weighing 40% of your body weight

Date					
Reps/ Weight/ Time/ Rounds					

#11 QUICK

WORKOUT

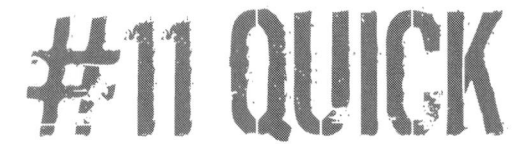

10 Sandbag Deadlifts
10 Sandbag Thrusters
10 Push Ups
10 Sandbag High Pulls

Aim to complete as many rounds as you can in 12 minutes.

MEASUREMENT

Record the total number of rounds you can complete in 12 minutes. Record the weight of the sandbag you used to complete this workout.

TARGET WEIGHT

Aim for a sandbag weighing 40% of your body weight

Date					
Reps/ Weight/ Time/ Rounds					

#12 QUICK

WORKOUT

20 seconds of work, 10 seconds of rest - repeat for a total of 8 working intervals. No rest between exercises.

Sandbag Shoulder Squats (switch shoulder each round)
Sandbag Thruster Burpees
Push Ups

MEASUREMENT

Record your total repetitions for the whole sequence. Record the weight of the sandbag you used to complete this workout.

TARGET WEIGHT

Aim for a sandbag weighing 30% of your body weight

Date					
Reps/ Weight/ Time/ Rounds					

Part 11: Quick Workouts

#13 QUICK

WORKOUT

5 Knees-to-Elbows
5 Sandbag Zercher Squats
5 Sandbag Push Jerks

Aim to complete as many rounds as you can in 12 minutes.

MEASUREMENT

Record the total number of rounds you can complete in 12 minutes. Record the weight of the sandbag you used to complete this workout.

TARGET WEIGHT

Aim for a sandbag weighing 50% of your body weight

Date					
Reps/ Weight/ Time/ Rounds					

#14 QUICK

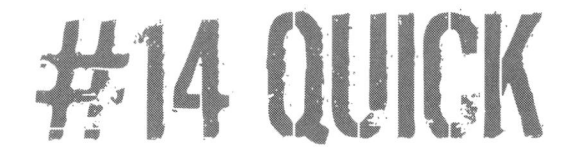

WORKOUT

10 Sandbag Bear Hug Squats
200m Run

Aim to complete as many rounds as you can in 12 minutes.

MEASUREMENT

Record the total number of rounds you can complete in 12 minutes. Record the weight of the sandbag you used to complete this workout.

TARGET WEIGHT

Aim for a sandbag weighing 50% of your body weight

Date					
Reps/ Weight/ Time/ Rounds					

#15 QUICK

WORKOUT

3 Pull Ups
6 Sandbag High Pulls
9 Sandbag Overhead Press
12 Body weight Squats

Aim to complete as many rounds as you can in 12 minutes.

MEASUREMENT

Record the total number of rounds you can complete in 12 minutes. Record the weight of the sandbag you used to complete this workout.

TARGET WEIGHT

Aim for a sandbag weighing 40% of your body weight

Date					
Reps/ Weight/ Time/ Rounds					

Part 11: Quick Workouts 183

#16 QUICK

WORKOUT

10 Sandbag Push Press
10 Box Jumps
10 Sandbag Cleans

Aim to complete as many rounds as you can in 15 minutes.

MEASUREMENT

Record the total number of rounds you can complete in 15 minutes. Record the weight of the sandbag you used to complete this workout.

TARGET WEIGHT

Aim for a sandbag weighing 40% of your body weight

Date					
Reps/ Weight/ Time/ Rounds					

#17 QUICK

WORKOUT

10 Sandbag Cleans
10 Sandbag Walking Lunges
10 Sandbag Thruster Burpees

Aim to complete as many rounds as you can in 15 minutes.

MEASUREMENT

Record the total number of rounds you can complete in 15 minutes. Record the weight of the sandbag you used to complete this workout.

TARGET WEIGHT

Aim for a sandbag weighing 40% of your body weight

Date					
Reps/ Weight/ Time/ Rounds					

#18 QUICK

WORKOUT

5 Sandbag Thrusters
50m Sandbag Load Carry
10 Sandbag Shoulders (5 each side)

Aim to complete as many rounds as you can in 15 minutes.

MEASUREMENT

Record the total number of rounds you can complete in 15 minutes. Record the weight of the sandbag you used to complete this workout.

TARGET WEIGHT

Aim for a sandbag weighing 40% of your body weight

Date					
Reps/ Weight/ Time/ Rounds					

#19 QUICK

WORKOUT

150 Skips
10 Pull Ups
10 Sandbag Floor Press

Aim to complete as many rounds as you can in 15 minutes.

MEASUREMENT

Record the total number of rounds you can complete in 15 minutes. Record the weight of the sandbag you used to complete this workout.

TARGET WEIGHT

Aim for a sandbag weighing 40% of your body weight

Date					
Reps/ Weight/ Time/ Rounds					

#20 QUICK

WORKOUT

3 Pull Ups
6 Sandbag Thrusters
9 Push Ups
12 Sandbag Jump Squats

Aim to complete as many rounds as you can in 15 minutes.

MEASUREMENT

Record the total number of rounds you can complete in 15 minutes. Record the weight of the sandbag you used to complete this workout.

TARGET WEIGHT

Aim for a sandbag weighing 50% of your body weight

Date					
Reps/ Weight/ Time/ Rounds					

PART 12
SANDBAG-ONLY WORKOUTS

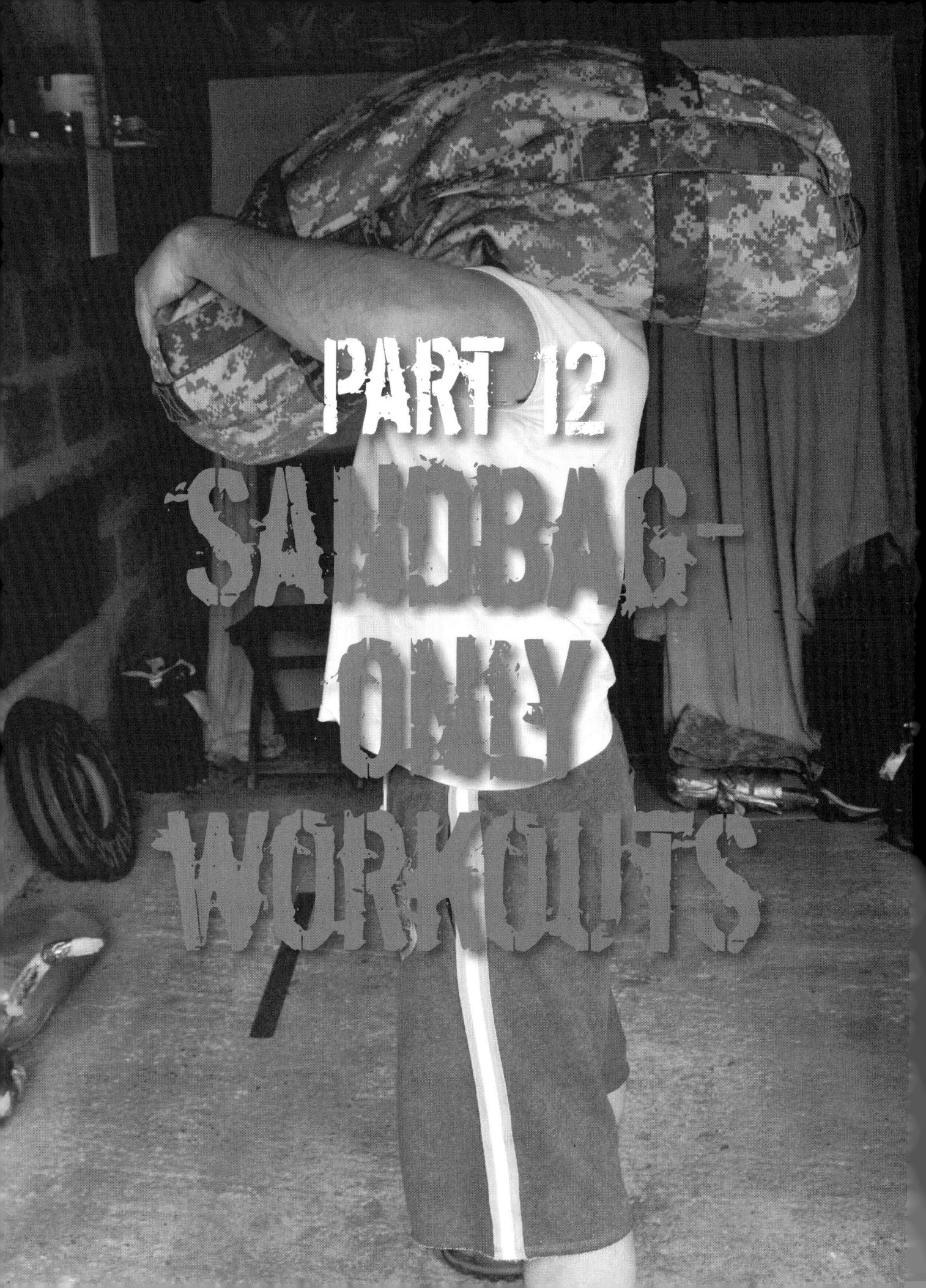

Sandbag

noun | sand·bag

1. A bag filled with sand and used in fortifications, as ballast, or as a weapon.

I'm a firm believer in the fact that a well rounded fitness training programme contains a range of elements and the use of whatever training tools are specific to your needs. At Sandbag Fitness we believe that a mastery of your own body weight (with exercises like Push Ups and Pull Ups) and the ability to control external loads (like the sandbag) are both important.

However, if you have nothing but a sandbag then these are the workouts for you.

SANDBAG-ONLY

"SANDBAGS HAVE BEEN LIFTED, LOADED, AND CARRIED FOR LONGER THAN WE HAVE ALL BEEN ALIVE. THERE IS SOMETHING TO BE SAID FOR ANY TOOL THAT STANDS THE ULTIMATE TEST OF TIME. SANDBAGS HAVE STUCK AROUND FOR A REASON. THEY WORK."

— ROSS ENAMAIT

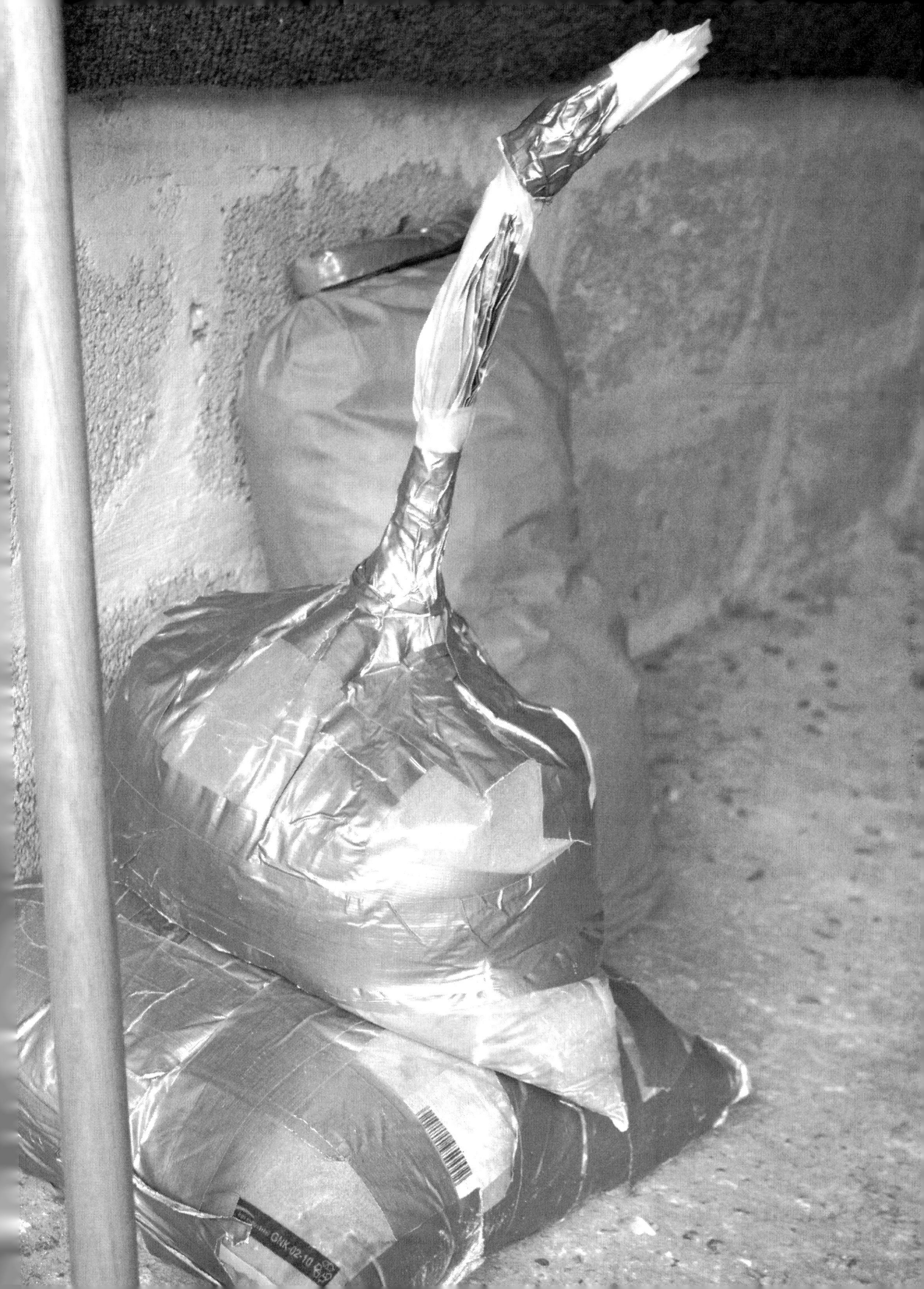

#1 SANDBAG-ONLY

WORKOUT

Sandbag Jump Squats, Sandbag Shoulder-to-Shoulder Press, Sandbag Snatches, Sandbag Overhead Press, Sandbag Zercher Squats.

Perform each exercise for 1 minute, giving a total round of 5 minutes. Record the number of repetitions performed within each minute for each exercise. There is a 1 minute rest period between each set of 5 exercises but a running clock during each round. Repeat for 3 rounds in total.

MEASUREMENT

Record your total repetitions for the whole sequence. Record the weight of the sandbag you used to complete this workout.

TARGET WEIGHT

Aim for a sandbag weighing 30% of your body weight

Date					
Reps/ Weight/ Time/ Rounds					

#2 SANDBAG-ONLY

WORKOUT

22 Sandbag Step Ups
22 Sandbag Shoulder-to-Shoulder Press
22 Sandbag Good Mornings

Repeat for a total of 6 rounds.

MEASUREMENT

Aim to complete the workout in as fast a time as you can. Record the weight of the sandbag you used to complete this workout.

TARGET WEIGHT

Aim for a sandbag weighing 30% of your body weight

Date					
Reps/ Weight/ Time/ Rounds					

#3 SANDBAG-ONLY

WORKOUT

20 seconds of work, 10 seconds of rest - repeat for a total of 8 working intervals. No rest between exercises.

Sandbag Round-the-Worlds (switch direction each interval)
Sandbag Walking Lunges
Sandbag High Pulls
Sandbag Snatches

MEASUREMENT

Record your total repetitions for the whole sequence. Record the weight of the sandbag you used to complete this workout.

TARGET WEIGHT

Aim for a sandbag weighing 30% of your body weight, 15% for the Round-the-Worlds

Date					
Reps/ Weight/ Time/ Rounds					

#4 SANDBAG-ONLY

WORKOUT

Sandbag Floor Press
Sandbag Bear Hug Squat

Every minute, on the minute. In minute 1 perform 1 repetition of each exercise, in minute 2 perform 2 repetitions of each exercise etc. Keep going until you can no longer complete the required repetitions.

MEASUREMENT

Record the number of rounds you can complete before reaching failure. Record the weight of the sandbag you used to complete this workout.

TARGET WEIGHT

Aim for a sandbag weighing 40% of your body weight

Date					
Reps/ Weight/ Time/ Rounds					

#5 SANDBAG-ONLY

WORKOUT

5 Sandbag Thruster Burpees
10 Sandbag Deadlifts
20 Sandbag Swings

Aim to complete as many rounds as you can in 30 minutes.

MEASUREMENT

Record the total number of rounds you can complete in 30 minutes. Record the weight of the sandbag you used to complete this workout.

TARGET WEIGHT

Aim for a sandbag weighing 30% of your body weight

Date					
Reps/ Weight/ Time/ Rounds					

#6 SANDBAG-ONLY

WORKOUT

Sandbag Front Squats, Sandbag Floor Press, Sandbag Bent-over-Row, Sandbag Get Ups, Sandbag Swings.

Perform each exercise for 1 minute, giving a total round of 5 minutes. Record the number of repetitions performed within each minute for each exercise. There is a 1 minute rest period between each set of 5 exercises but a running clock during each round. Repeat for 3 rounds in total.

MEASUREMENT

Record your total repetitions for the whole sequence. Record the weight of the sandbag you used to complete this workout.

TARGET WEIGHT

Aim for a sandbag weighing 30% of your body weight

Date					
Reps/ Weight/ Time/ Rounds					

#7 SANDBAG-ONLY

WORKOUT

20 seconds of work, 10 seconds of rest - repeat for a total of 8 working intervals. No rest between exercises.

Sandbag Cleans
Sandbag Shoulder-to-Shoulder Press
Sandbag Walking Lunges (switch sides each interval)

MEASUREMENT

Record your total repetitions for the whole sequence. Record the weight of the sandbag you used to complete this workout.

TARGET WEIGHT

Aim for a sandbag weighing 40% of your body weight

Date					
Reps/ Weight/ Time/ Rounds					

#8 SANDBAG-ONLY

WORKOUT

100 Sandbag Floor Press
75 Sandbag Zercher Squats
50 Sandbag Shoulder Get Ups (25 each side)

Complete as fast as you can in this order - reps can be broken up into sets where necessary.

MEASUREMENT

Aim to complete the workout in as fast a time as you can. Record the weight of the sandbag you used to complete this workout.

TARGET WEIGHT

Aim for a sandbag weighing 40% of your body weight

Date					
Reps/ Weight/ Time/ Rounds					

200 Part 12: Sandbag-Only Workouts

#9 SANDBAG-ONLY

WORKOUT

10 Sandbag Bear Hug Step Ups (5 each side)
10 Sandbag Thrusters
20m Sandbag Drag

Rest for 1 - 2 minutes and repeat for a total of 5 rounds.

MEASUREMENT

Aim to complete the workout in as fast a time as you can. Record the weight of the sandbag you used to complete this workout.

TARGET WEIGHT

Aim for a sandbag weighing 60% of your body weight

Date					
Reps/ Weight/ Time/ Rounds					

#10 SANDBAG-ONLY

WORKOUT

10 Sandbag Bear Hug Squat
100m Sandbag Load Carry
10 Sandbag Shoulders (5 each side)

Repeat for a total of 5 rounds.

MEASUREMENT

Aim to complete the workout in as fast a time as you can. Record the weight of the sandbag you used to complete this workout.

TARGET WEIGHT

Aim for a sandbag weighing 50% of your body weight

Date					
Reps/ Weight/ Time/ Rounds					

PART 13
CHALLENGE WORKOUTS

Challenge

noun | chal·lenge

1. To confront or defy boldly.
2. To call out to duel or combat.
3. To invite into competition.

While all of the workouts listed in this guide are challenging, the following section details a range of workouts that I've developed to work as standalone challenges. Some have been developed specifically for sandbag training while others are adapted from existing tests that exist within the Military, CrossFit and Professional Sports. As with all of the other workouts you can use these as benchmarks to chart your progress.

The sessions also work particularly well with a partner or small group. Train hard!

Part 13: Challenge Workouts

CHALLENGE

"IMPOSSIBLE IS NOT A FACT. IT'S AN OPINION. IMPOSSIBLE IS NOT A DECLARATION. IT'S A DARE. IMPOSSIBLE IS POTENTIAL. IMPOSSIBLE IS TEMPORARY. IMPOSSIBLE IS NOTHING."

MUHAMMAD ALI

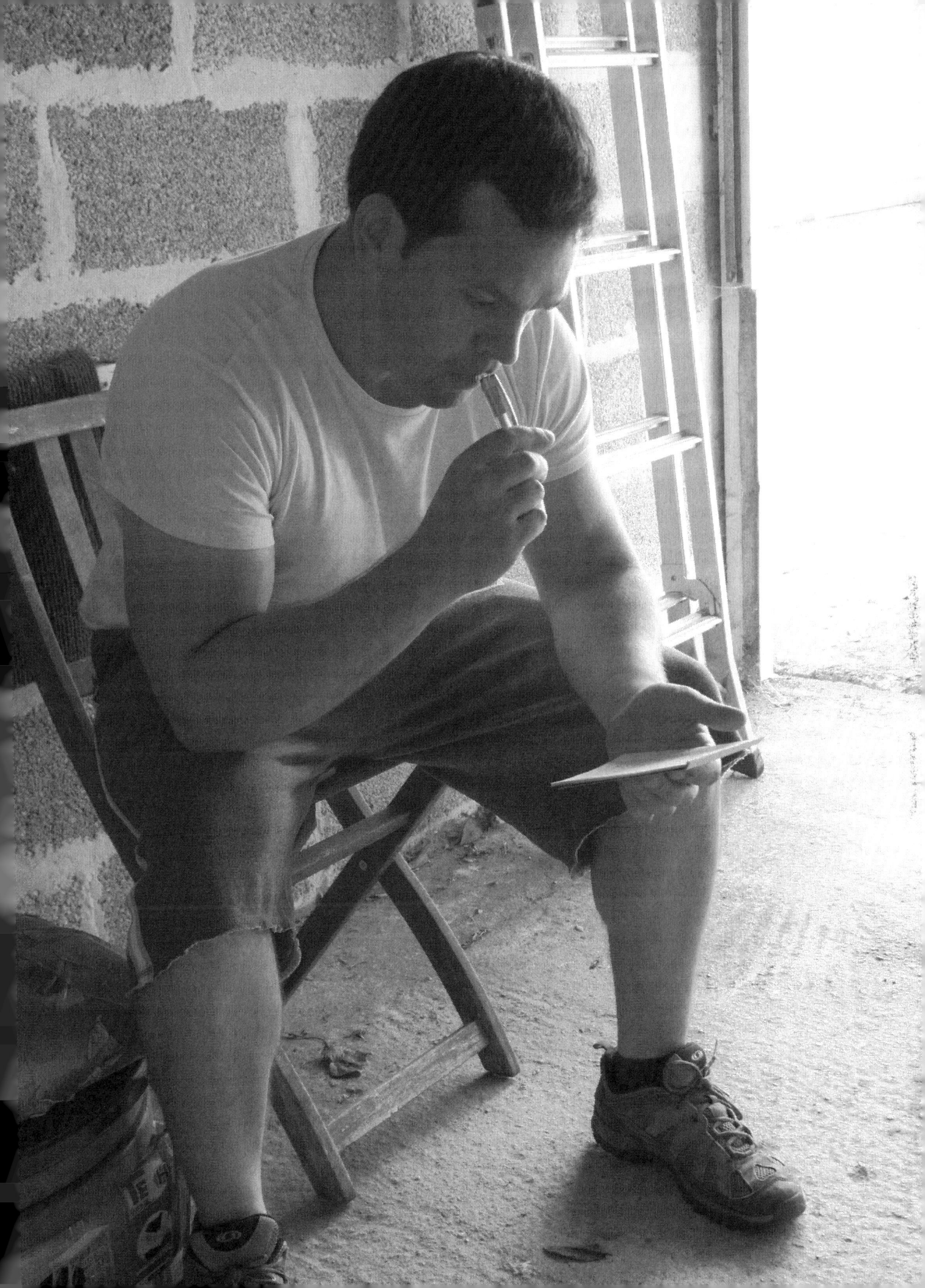

206 Part 13: Challenge Workouts

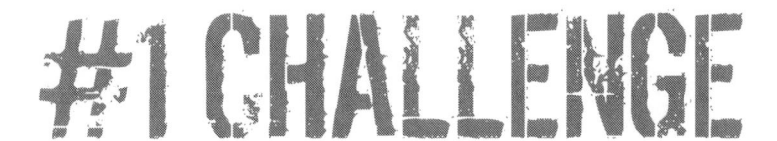

#1 CHALLENGE

WORKOUT

Sandbag Fitness Bronze Workout

20 Sandbag Deadlift
20 Sandbag Back Squat
20 Sandbag Shoulders (10 each side)
15 Sandbag High Pull
15 Sandbag Overhead Press
15 Sandbag Floor Press
20 Sandbag Walking Lunge (10 each side)
5 Sandbag Shoulder Get Ups (each side)

MEASUREMENT

Aim to complete the workout in 10 minutes or less.

TARGET WEIGHT

Aim for a sandbag weighing 40% of your body weight

Date					
Reps/ Weight/ Time/ Rounds					

#2 CHALLENGE

WORKOUT

Sandbag Fitness Silver Workout

50 Sandbag Clean & Press

MEASUREMENT

Aim to complete the workout in 15 minutes or less.

TARGET WEIGHT

Aim for a sandbag weighing 100% of your body weight

Date					
Reps/ Weight/ Time/ Rounds					

#3 CHALLENGE

WORKOUT

The Sandbag Mile

Set out a course of 1 mile. Carry your sandbag any way you wish over the course.

MEASUREMENT

Aim to complete the workout in 12 minutes or less.

TARGET WEIGHT

Aim for a sandbag weighing 50% of your body weight

Date					
Reps/ Weight/ Time/ Rounds					

#4 CHALLENGE

WORKOUT

The Sandbag Milo of Croton Experiment

Start off with a sandbag weighing approximately 50% of your body weight. On day 1 perform a single Sandbag Clean & Press. On day 2 add an additional 1-2 lbs of weight and perform a single Sandbag Clean & Press. Repeat each day until you can no longer add any additional weight.

MEASUREMENT

TARGET WEIGHT

Start with a sandbag weighing 50% of your body weight, aim to reach a sandbag weighing 150%+ of your body weight

Date					
Reps/ Weight/ Time/ Rounds					

#5 CHALLENGE

WORKOUT

NHL Combine Test - modified

This is adapted from a NHL Combine Test. Instead of using the Bench Press we'll be using the Sandbag Overhead Press exercise. Set a metronome at a rate of 25 per minute, each click signifying either a press or a return of the sandbag to the chest. Perform the test until you can no longer maintain the required timing.

MEASUREMENT

0-5 repetitions is poor; 6-10 repetitions is average; 11-15 repetitions is good; 15-24 repetitions is very good; 25+ repetitions is excellent

TARGET WEIGHT

Aim for a sandbag weighing 50% of your body weight

Date					
Reps/ Weight/ Time/ Rounds					

#6 CHALLENGE

WORKOUT

USMC Ammo Can Lift - modified

This is adapted from a United States Marine Corps fitness test. Instead of using an ammo can, we'll be using another awkward object for the test - your sandbag. This test utilises the Sandbag Overhead Press exercise.

MEASUREMENT

The maximum score for males is 91 repetitions; the maximum score for females is 61 repetitions. The test commences when you perform your first repetition. The test ends when you can no longer complete repetitions or need to drop the sandbag.

TARGET WEIGHT

Aim for a sandbag weighing 30lbs

Date					
Reps/ Weight/ Time/ Rounds					

212 Part 13: Challenge Workouts

#7 CHALLENGE

WORKOUT

CrossFit Sandbag 'Grace' - modified

30 Sandbag Clean & Press

MEASUREMENT

Aim to complete the workout in 4 minutes or less.

TARGET WEIGHT

Aim for a sandbag weighing 135lbs

Date					
Reps/ Weight/ Time/ Rounds					

#8 CHALLENGE

WORKOUT

CrossFit Sandbag 'Fran' - modified

21 - 15 - 9 of the following exercises (perform 21 repetitions of each one, then 15, and then 9):

Sandbag Thruster
Pull Ups

MEASUREMENT

Aim to complete the workout in 5 minutes or less.

TARGET WEIGHT

Aim for a sandbag weighing 95lbs

Date					
Reps/ Weight/ Time/ Rounds					

#9 CHALLENGE

WORKOUT

CrossFit Sandbag 'Randy' - modified

75 Sandbag Power Cleans

MEASUREMENT

Aim to complete the workout in 5 minutes or less.

TARGET WEIGHT

Aim for a sandbag weighing 75lbs

Date					
Reps/ Weight/ Time/ Rounds					

#10 CHALLENGE

WORKOUT

CrossFit Sandbag 'Danny' - modified

30 Box Jumps
20 Sandbag Push Press
30 Pull Ups

Aim to complete as many rounds as you can in 20 minutes.

MEASUREMENT

Aim to complete 5 rounds in 20 minutes.

TARGET WEIGHT

Aim for a sandbag weighing 115lbs

Date					
Reps/ Weight/ Time/ Rounds					

AFTERWORD

Health and fitness is a lifelong pursuit and I hope this guide has gone a long way to providing you with the means to make significant changes to both. It can be difficult to stay focused on the week to week work required and I know that many people struggle with this aspect of training. They start with good intentions but then life gets in the way.

Having been at this for 20 years now I can say one thing with certainty - while your abilities can change, the ability to give your all does not. Your all is of course always there, ready to be accessed. While your strength and fitness changes over time you'll always have the ability to pick up your sandbag and leave everything on the table. There is great power in that and I urge you to always stay focused on the reward that comes from the journey and not just the destination.

If you do manage to get through all of the workouts in this guide, and log multiple performances for each one, then you will undoubtedly be head and shoulders above those around you. You'll have learned more about your body, and your ability to push yourself, than you could ever get from simply reading the book.

WHILE YOUR ABILITIES CAN CHANGE, THE ABILITY TO GIVE YOUR ALL DOES NOT.

FAQ

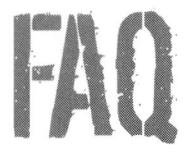

I can't hit the Target Weight for the workout. What should I do?
This is not a problem at all. The target weight is provided as a guide for you to aim for. If you aren't yet at that stage where you are able to lift that much weight in your sandbag then start lighter and work towards it. Likewise, you shouldn't necessarily ease up if you can achieve the target weight for a workout. Aim high!

I can't perform things like Pull Ups or Push Ups. What should I do?
Scale back the exercise to make it more appropriate for you. For Push Ups this might mean performing Incline Push Ups or Push Ups from the knees. Likewise with Pull Ups, Body Rows or Jumping Pull Ups are a good transition exercise. When it comes to questions of this nature you should consider the exercise as a variant.

The workouts are too easy for me. How can I make them harder?
All of the workouts can be made more challenging by adding more weight, going faster or completing more repetitions. How you modify the workout will be dependent on your specific goals. You can also experiment with adding additional rounds or time to the workouts.

I have an injury. Can I follow these workouts?
As with all injuries you should ensure that you are recovered enough to tackle a programme of exercise and activity. I advise that you seek guidance from a medical professional if you are unsure of the suitability of any of the workouts in this guide.

How many times per week should I do these workouts?
It does depend on the specific workouts that you are doing and also on the other activity that you're performing during the week. As a general rule 2-4 training sessions per week is sufficient for continued progress.

If I can't complete a full round in my remaining time, what should I do?
Do a partial round. If you can only manage a single repetition of an exercise in the next round before you run out of time then that's ok. In fact, that's the best strategy for chipping away at targets of this nature - just aim to do a little bit more of the required work each time.

I've finished all of the workouts? What now?
Firstly I advise you to complete each workout at least 5 times, aiming to improve your performance each time. I'd honestly be very surprised to hear from anyone who manages to do this but if that happens then drop me an email - I'd be more than happy to go through some additional programming for you.

I can't lift as much weight in a sandbag as I can with a barbell - is that a problem?
The sandbag won't cooperate quite as much as a barbell, and that's ok. So it's perfectly normal that you won't be able to lift as much weight in a sandbag. As such it's well suited to workouts that are more geared towards athletic conditioning. If your primary goal is strength then I'd advise a combination of some sandbag training and some barbell training.

Should I follow a specific diet with these workouts?
The book Sandbag Fitness: Lean & Strong goes into more detail regarding my recommended dietary practices. In general I advise a diet that contains plenty of protein and fat, fruit and vegetables and unprocessed foods.

WANT TO LEARN MORE?

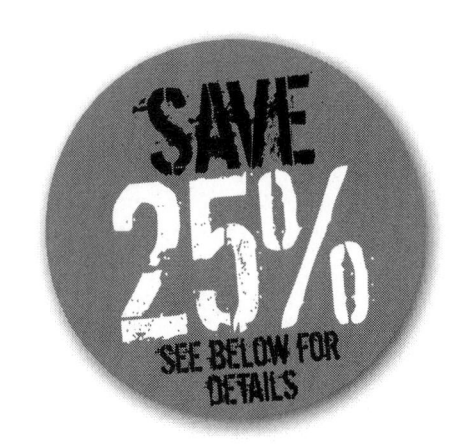

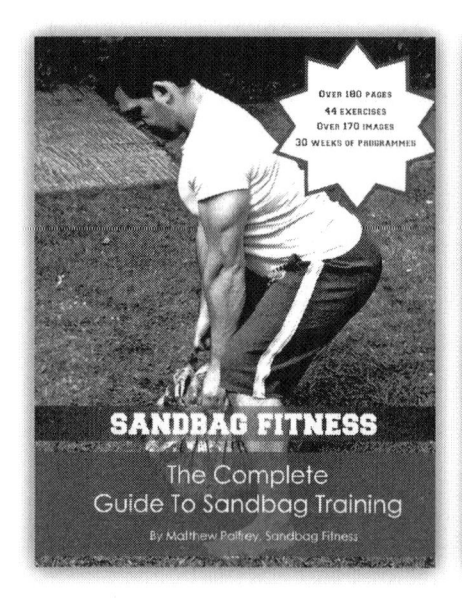

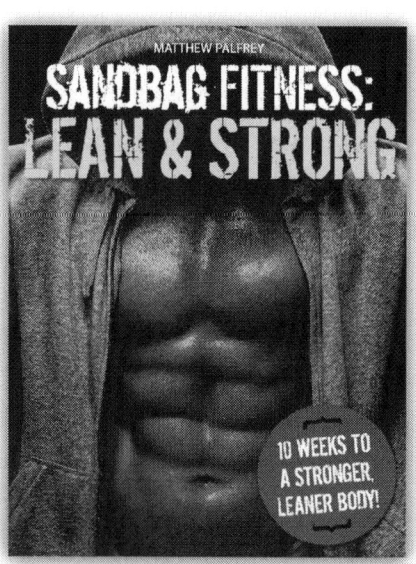

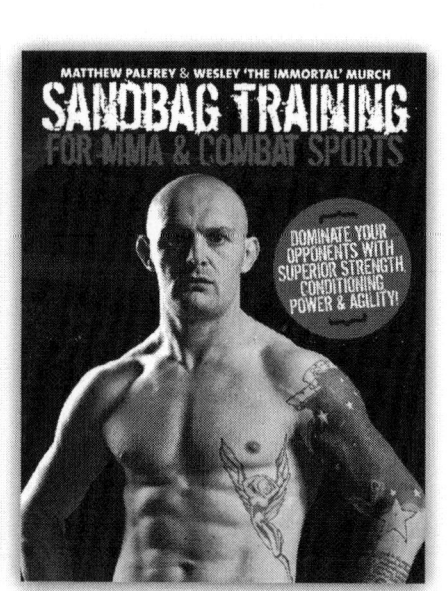

If you've enjoyed this book why not purchase The Complete Guide To Sandbag Training, Sandbag Training For MMA & Combat Sports or Sandbag Fitness: Lean & Strong. All three books are packed with training programmes aimed at improving your strength and conditioning.

And you can use the discount code **sandbagfitness25** to get 25% off now!

www.sandbagfitnessstore.com

MATTHEW PALFREY

The Sandbag Fitness Blog is packed full of workouts, tips, advice and sandbag training information.

Matthew Palfrey on Facebook https://www.facebook.com/mattpalfrey

Sandbag Fitness Blog

http://sandbagfitnessstore.com/blogs/sandbag-fitness-blog

Sandbag Fitness on Facebook https://www.facebook.com/sandbagfitness

Sandbag Fitness on Twitter https://twitter.com/sandbagfit

Sandbag Fitness on Pinterest

http://pinterest.com/matthewpalfrey/sandbag-fitness

Sandbag Fitness on Youtube http://www.youtube.com/user/CoachPalfrey

Sandbag Fitness Store http://sandbagfitnessstore.com

ACKNOWLEDGEMENTS

As always, there are far too many people to mention in my acknowledgements. And in many ways my greatest thanks go to those who don't know that they should be here. Unknowing sounding boards, friends and family, colleagues, customers and competitors.

Particular thanks go to Brute Force Sandbags who continue to support me with the best sandbag training equipment available.

But anyone that knows me well also knows that I do it all for Ali. Without her support not only would it not be possible, but I'd lose my greatest motivation.

MATTHEW PALFREY

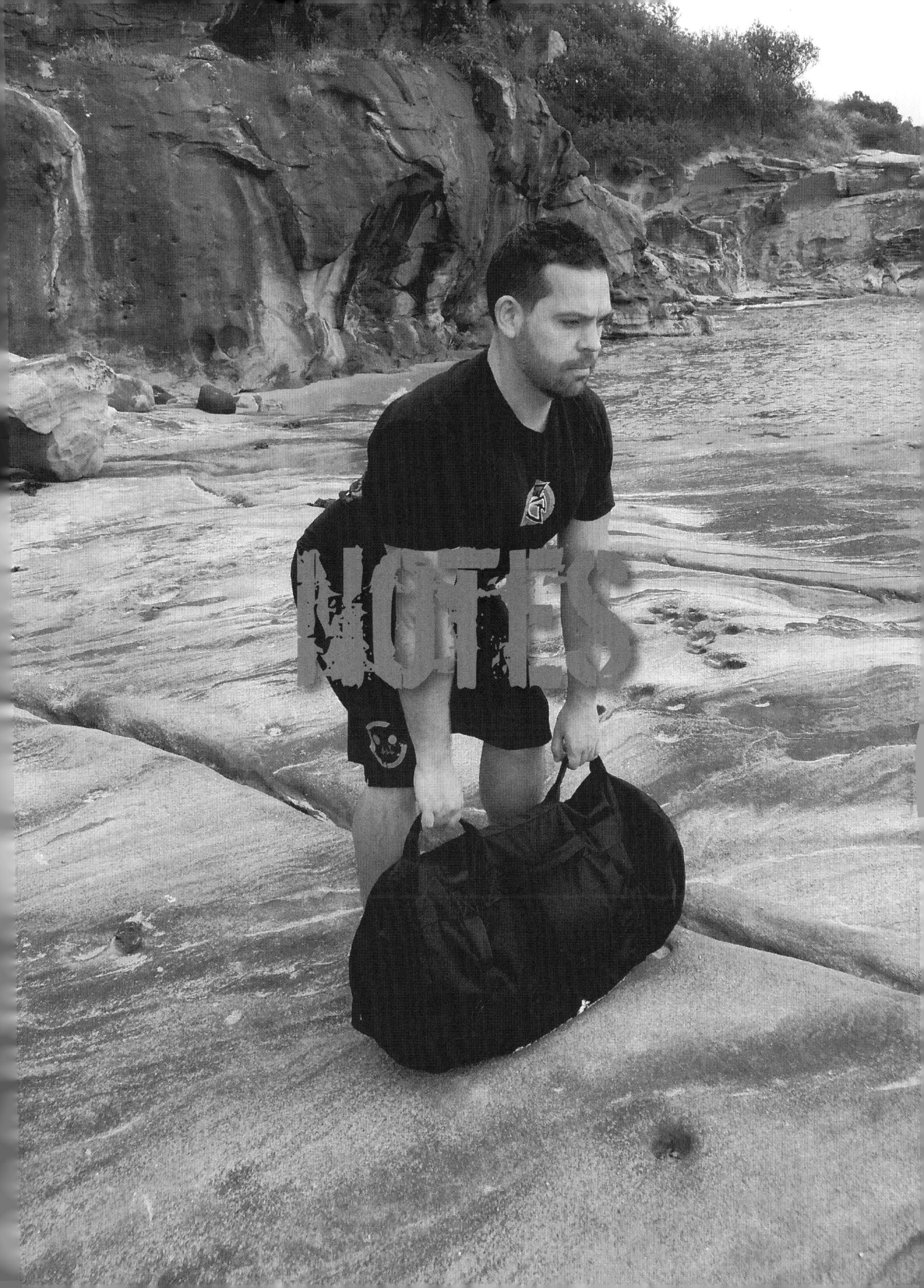

NOTES

NOTES

NOTES